Bedtime Stories for Insomniacs

Surprisingly Original Sleep Tips from
The Effortless Sleep Method
Good Sleepers' Club

By Sasha Stephens,
Author of The Effortless Sleep Method

Dark Moon Ltd

GW00645361

AUTHOR'S NOTE: The techniques, ideas, and opinions here are not intended as a substitute for proper medical advice. The information provided here is solely for informational purposes only. All information is generalised, presented for informational purposes only, not medical advice, and not to rely on this information as medical advice and to consult a qualified medical, dietary, fitness or other appropriate professional for their specific needs. This information has not been evaluated by any government agency and the information is not intended to 'diagnose, treat, cure or prevent any disease'. Any application of the techniques, ideas, and suggestions here are at the reader's sole discretion and risk. The author and the publisher expressly disclaim responsibility for any adverse effects arising from following this advice.

While every effort has been made to ensure reliability and accuracy of the information within, all liability, negligence or otherwise, from any use, misuse or abuse of the operation of any methods, strategies, instructions or ideas contained in the material herein, is the sole responsibility of the reader.

Published by Dark Moon Ltd in 2013
Copyright © 2013 Sasha Stephens. All rights reserved.

The author and publisher of this material make no medical claims for its use. This material is not intended to treat, diagnose nor cure any illness. If you need medical attention, please consult your doctor.

Cover designer: Michael Warren

A CIP catalogue record for this book
is available from the British Library.

First Edition

ISBN: 978-0-9571-0482-2

Bedtime Stories
for Insomniacs

Also by Sasha Stephens

The Effortless Sleep Method

The Effortless Sleep Companion

To My Readers

What Is
The Effortless Sleep Method?

The 12 promises of the *Effortless Sleep Method* comprise a common-sense, non-drug approach to beating long-term, chronic insomnia. It has frequently been described as 'ground-breaking' by doctors, therapists and ex-insomniacs alike.

The method works so well precisely because it has *not* been created by a doctor, but by someone who has *been there, done that*, and who knows intimately the thought processes that go on in the mind of the insomniac.

Part sleep hygiene, part cognitive therapy, and part pep-talk, both *The Effortless Sleep Method* and its follow-up book, *The Effortless Sleep Companion*, have proved to be astonishingly successful in helping chronic insomniacs get their lives back.

Why 'Bedtime Stories'? Are They to Be Read Only at Bedtime?

The Good Sleepers' Club was the name given to those people who were following or had followed *The Effortless Sleep Method* for insomnia. Completely unlike many online sleep support sites and insomnia forums, The Good Sleepers' Club had only a positive message. It did not set out to scare or intimidate. It did not exist for the purposes of commiseration or even sympathy. The philosophy of the Good Sleepers' Club was the same as that of *The Effortless Sleep Method* – a no-nonsense, straightforward, tell-it-like-it-is approach to beating insomnia. My intention was that even the most desperate of insomniacs would feel less alone, where they were in company with recovering insomniacs like themselves.

For some years, I kept in constant touch by email with the club, sending out almost daily motivational emails, just to remind members that someone was still here for the. Called *Bedtime Stories*, these were short, snappy messages, intended to keep you on track with following The Effortless Sleep Method. *Bedtime Stories* are little snippets of sleepy wisdom, written to inspire, empower and remind you to keep on track with good sleep. Sometimes loving, sometimes harsh, always truthful.

Many people came to really look forward and to depend on these sleep tips and many times I was asked to collate them all in a book.

This book is a response to that request. While it does not contain *every* tip I have ever sent, it does contain a carefully selected number of some of the most popular ones. They have been intentionally arranged in *no particular order* to prevent your flicking just to the sections which seem relevant to your particular situation (and so risking missing out on loads of helpful advice you may otherwise have overlooked). And in answer to the title question… you can read them at *any* time of day or night.

Although you will doubtless find this book helpful in its own right, bear in mind that it has been written as a *support*, not as a *replacement* for following the 12 promises of the Method itself (listed on page 8).

For this reason, I highly recommend that you read this book in conjunction with either or both of my other books *The Effortless Sleep Method* and *The Effortless Sleep Companion*.

Warning: *Bedtime Stories* are only for those seriously committed to becoming good sleepers. I want to get you sleeping, *really* well. So be warned, I tell it like it is and do not mince my words. Because I don't just want to give you good sleep, I want to make you sleep better than you have ever done.

I Just Sneaked a Look at the 12 Promises. Do I Need to Read the Rest of the Book?

Taken in isolation, these 12 promises may not appear to be particularly different, effective or original. You may even have seen a couple of these instructions before in other sleep books.

But you need to realise that these 12 promises are just a tiny taste – a fraction of what the method has to offer. It is *never* by simply following the 12 promises that a person will come to cure their insomnia; it is by understanding the importance of each promise, what it does and why it works.

The real magic of this programme lies in the changes that will occur *within you* as you read these three books. My intention is not just to give you a set of instructions; it is to facilitate a shift in your thinking, understanding and beliefs – a shift which allows you to control, dominate and completely erase insomnia from your life.

The Method is not just 12 promises; it is an entire mind-set. The sum total of my knowledge of how to create this mind-set is contained in my three books.

You've Still Got It...

Somewhere, perhaps hidden deep down inside you, is the innate, primordial ability to sleep perfectly, deeply, effortlessly, like a child.

All that's stopping you from accessing that delicious, sleepy perfection are the years of baggage, the bad memories, repeated negativity and obsessive thoughts which have piled up.

Just *have faith* that this is true. Just *have faith* that deep-down *you can sleep perfectly.*

If it's difficult to get a grasp of this right now, just try it, imagine it, try it on for size. Humour me. Humour yourself!

You may *just* get a message through to that hidden, childlike quality to let it know it's safe to come out and play.

And when good sleep shows itself, don't ask where it's been all this time, don't demand to know how long it's going to stay. Just be really, really happy that it's here.

In this way, it may just want to come out to play more often.

Anomalies Welcome

Don't let doctors, therapists, family members or friends make you unusual, different, like a freak. Just because someone is bemused by your problem, or shocked by its severity, or outright doesn't believe you, this doesn't mean you aren't normal!

You are in good company here at the Good Sleepers' Club, because unlike your doctor, therapist, friends and family, everyone here knows how it feels to struggle with insomnia.

Whatever you feel, however terrible, strange or unusual your problem, I have no doubt heard it before, *and worse*. Take it from one who knows, take it from one who has seen it happen, again and again…*you are normal*, and you *can get better*…

…from even the very worst insomnia.

Choose Your Idols Carefully

It's very strange...the way we always tend to identify with those whose insomnia is far worse than our own. We hear a tale of someone never recovering, of going mad, of *dying* of insomnia, and all we can think is that the same must be in store for us. Why do we do this? We know *nothing* about this person. We know nothing about their life, their history, their character, their general mental state. Why on earth suppose we have *anything* in common with them?

I'll give you someone to identify with: try identifying with Maya, who wrote to me yesterday to tell me that after *fifty* years of chronic insomnia, she is now making real progress. Or identify with James, who wrote a few days ago to tell me he feels happier and more positive than he has ever done in his life. After all, you are following the same programme as these people, you are getting the same support as these people, you are in the same *club* as these people. In fact, you have *loads* more in common with these success stories than you do with all those misery-mongers.

The truth is, career insomniacs and misery-mongers are not allowed in the Good Sleepers' Club.

The Promises of
The Effortless Sleep Method

1. Get less time in Bed

2. No naps

3. Get out of bed when you can't sleep

4. Get up at the same time every day

5. Do nothing in bed but sleep or have sex

6. Reduce or eliminate the pills

7. Stop clockwatching

8. Replace negative sleep talk with positive statements

9. Let go of the search for a miracle cure

10. Discover a relaxation technique that works for you

11. Decide on a safety thought

12. Put your life first

For more details, please read *The Effortless Sleep Method* or *The Effortless Sleep Companion.*

The Three Fundamentals Steps
to Curing Insomnia

1. Instil good sleep hygiene

2. Work on reducing tension

3. Replace negative thoughts and statements with positive ones

Is that it?

In short, yes. In basic terms, this is all you have to do to overcome even long-term chronic insomnia. Each of these three steps is covered by one or more of the 12 promises of The Effortless Sleep Method.

Unfortunately, the details are a *little* more complicated, so *read on…!*

Good Hygiene Is Essential for All

Don't make the mistake of assuming sleep hygiene won't work with a problem as bad as yours. Don't assume that because you have had no luck so far that such things just 'don't work for you'.

Sleep hygiene (summed up in the first seven promises) works to increase tiredness, to instil a routine and to create a new positive habit. Sleep hygiene works to increase *expectation* of sleep, to make the association of bed and sleep so strong that its effect can be overpowering – often allowing you to fall asleep rapidly and automatically.

So why hasn't it worked for you in the past?

Well, if you were not *also* attending to negative thinking and unhelpful beliefs, it's little wonder that sleep hygiene didn't have much of an effect. The force of negative beliefs is often so strong it can keep you awake through anything, even overpowering the strongest of sleeping pills. The benefit of sleep hygiene can thus often be lost behind a wall of fear, panic and negative thoughts about sleep. *This* is why many people come to believe that sleep hygiene is simply ineffective or irrelevant for them. It isn't. Not ever.

No, sleep hygiene alone won't cure most long-term insomniacs. But it is essential *for everyone*, to lay the foundations for the other promises to work their magic. And one thing is certain: you will find it almost impossible to overcome chronic insomnia if your sleep hygiene remains poor.

Insomnia Doesn't Exist

What is insomnia? Is it a disease, a condition an affliction? Or is it a monster, a demon, a curse?

It's none of these things. In fact … there is no such thing as insomnia.

What I mean is that insomniacs are not a different breed of person; they do not 'have' a condition which marks them out as incurable or ill.

I use the terms 'insomnia' and 'insomniac' because it's difficult to make myself understood without them, but I sometimes wonder whether it's possible to eliminate these terms from my writing.

Because in a very real sense, you do not *have* anything. This 'condition' does not exist in its own right. 'Insomnia' is just a word we give to some nights when we didn't sleep well. By applying a name, a label (especially a medical-sounding label) we make it real, give it credibility, importance. It then assumes a large and very real place in our lives.

If we could ban the use of the word 'insomnia', suddenly that monster doesn't seem so strong, so important, and a lot of its power drains away. Insomnia is a big fat nothing. Let's not give it any more importance. It doesn't deserve it.

What Are Affirmations?

Affirmations are just little repeated positive statements which provide a disciplined way to make sure that for at least part of the day, your sleep talk is in the right direction. I highly recommend that you use positive affirmations regularly.

Pick something you would like to be true, the *belief* that you think a really good sleeper would have. *A belief that would allow you to sleep.* It could be 'I'm still a *great* sleeper under all this', 'I trust that I can sleep really well', 'I *can* control my thoughts', 'I can sleep right through the night.' If you have sleep-maintenance insomnia, try 'I'm sleeping through much better these days.' These can slowly be upped in 'intensity' until you really do believe you are a world-champion sleeper.

If you are very anxious, affirmations can sometimes work to keep you reminded of your problem. In this case, try using less sleep-based ones such as 'I feel so calm/relaxed/centred.' Just the affirmation 'Life is good' or 'I am so happy' can work wonders.

Make sure your affirmation is framed in the positive (no 'nots', no 'don'ts') Stick it on Post-it® notes all over the house, and begin to repeat it *out loud*. When you say it, say it *with feeling*; really feel the meaning of the words. *Just mere repetition is pointless*; you must try to feel it, believe it. Sometimes, put the accent on different parts of the sentence: 'I'm still a *great* sleeper', or 'I'm *still* a great sleeper.'

Try saying it to yourself in the mirror – this is really tough but is extra-effective. Say your affirmation(s) about ten times, at least six times a day. You cannot do this too much. A funny thing will very quickly happen: your mind will start looking for things to make it true and focusing on them. Soon, it won't sound like a lie any more, and before you know it *it will be true*. Believe me, *this is how all beliefs are formed – repeated thought.*

Falling in Love with Sleep

If you find your bed is a place of misery and fear, it's time to rekindle your romance with bedtime.

Start the relationship afresh. Starch the sheets, light some candles, buy a new pillow. Think of all the things you love about your bed, and put all those niggling complaints aside. Find a way to look forward to bedtime, to love it.

Sounds silly and superficial doesn't it? Sounds like I have made up a trivial and trite little story for Valentine's Day.

It's not silly, and it works. Concentrate on all you love about bedtime, and that love will blossom.

Change Is the Only Constant

Do you have *really* negative thinking, worse than anyone? *I remember that.* No control over your thoughts at all? *That's what we all think.* Just can't cope with a missed night, no matter how important you know it is? *I've been there.* Think nothing is changing, that positive thinking doesn't work on you? *Yup, that too.*

Do you think I *haven't* had all these thoughts? Do you think I just switched on the positive thinking and instantly lit up like a paragon of spiritual loveliness? Whatever negative thought you've had, whatever crazy reaction, whatever ingrained belief, I've probably had it, felt it… got over it.

But it takes time. It doesn't happen straight away. And the first step is realising, accepting, believing, that no matter how bad or different it seems for you, we have all been there, *all this can change*, and that *you can do this*.

What IS a Safety Thought?

A safety thought is just my phrase for a 'safe thought' – a *fact*, something true that has happened, or something you believe, which calms and soothes you when you are worried about whether you will sleep. This might be along the lines of 'I can have a good day tomorrow even if I don't sleep' or 'I slept last Wednesday when I didn't expect to, so I can do the same tonight.'

When the panic comes over you and thoughts of not sleeping fill your head, you simply need to remind yourself of your safety thought.

Can you remember a night, or a stretch of nights when you slept really well? Can you remember a time when you didn't expect to sleep and yet still did? Try to find a comforting and encouraging *fact* about your sleep. Have you had even *one* good night's sleep recently? Pick whatever positive fact you feel would be most likely to give you hope. When you lie down at night, relax into the comfort of your safety thought and let it soothe you.

Just the Right Level of Discipline

One of my clients, David, is concerned that by following a programme like *The Effortless Sleep Method*, he is only adding to his obsession. He asked whether the following would be a good alternative course of action for a new insomniac...

"Rather than obsessively following any sort of programme or guidelines, perhaps you should sleep whenever you want and for as long or as little as you want. Perhaps you should lie in bed in the mornings and nap during the day. If you want to sleep, *just sleep*. Have no idea what your 'normal getting up' time is, nor how long you spend in bed. Every day will be different. In this way, perhaps your obsession will dissolve and so will your insomnia."

Sorry. It doesn't work.

If we lived in a world where it never much mattered when we got up, or whether we slept, or where we never had precise calls on our time, this sort of sleeping pattern might not be such a problem. But we don't roll into work at 11.30 am, we arrange to see our friend at 6pm, not 'when we feel like it', and flights leave on time; they do not wait for us to have had enough sleep!

For these reasons (and plenty of others), a *slightly* harsher regime is always needed – *at least in the beginning*.

It's the Worry That's the Killer

You know... sometimes I still have a less than perfect night. The amazing thing is, I am now able to miss nights quite easily. I get up feeling rough, but after a coffee* and some food I feel better. By lunchtime I have usually forgotten I had even missed a night's sleep!

This seems incredible when I think of how it used to affect me. A missed night's sleep would once have sent me into a pit of depression, even creating physical symptoms such as tummy aches and a sore throat. Now I just shrug it off. This is what has made me realise that it's the fear, the tension and the worry that's the real killer, not the lack of sleep *per se*.

*Sometimes I need two coffees.

Creating Associations

On a recent holiday in Brittany, I spent a lot of time being driven around in the back of a Prius. It turns out that the back seat of a Prius is really rather comfortable! I fell asleep twice on the five hour drive to the town where we were staying, and then again while driving the following day.

Having created this association, I found myself falling asleep every time I got in the car, even on short trips. No matter how hard I tried, I literally couldn't stay awake.

This just reminds me of the importance of the sleep hygiene rules, particularly those which are designed to create a strong association of bed and sleep.

I know these rules are a drag, but stick with them. When an association is strong enough, you really can find yourself falling asleep within seconds of lying down... without even thinking about it.

The Dreaded Promise 3

Everyone hates promise 3: "Get out of bed when you can't sleep."

Now, I am not saying that you should get out of bed after twenty minutes, or half an hour or any such arbitrary time. The only promise you must make is that you get up once you are wide awake. In fact, if you have lain there for an hour, but still feel nice and drowsy and sleepy, like you could still fall asleep, it is probably better to stay where you are, *sleep may still come*.

But if you are becoming wide awake and stressed, get up.

Every minute that you lie in bed wide awake strengthens the association of bed and being awake. You want the very act of getting into bed to start inducing sleep. This is how some people claim to 'fall asleep as soon as their head hits the pillow'. These people don't have any special ability – they just have an incredibly strong association between bed and sleep. Now, you *can* create just such a trigger, but *not* if you lie around in bed not sleeping.

Also, many people are more likely to fall asleep very shortly after getting into bed. If you go to bed, nice and sleepy, and then find that you have become awake again, it can take a very long time for the sleepy feeling to return *if you remain in bed*.

If you get out of bed, you can start the whole falling asleep process all over again much more quickly.

This move seems to work best in the earlier part of the night, and is less effective closer to getting up time. If you wake at say, 5am, I wouldn't bother with getting up before your alarm goes off at 7. Just enjoy the rest for a couple of hours.

And for most people, getting up once or twice is enough. If I had been up twice in a night, for example, I wouldn't bother with getting up a third time.

Discipline is good, but torture is not. I don't expect you to go through hell in following my advice.

Remember the Night When...

…you slept like a baby, against all the odds? You know the one… that night where all the circumstances were wrong, when you thought there was not a chance in hell of your sleeping…and yet you did?

Felt good didn't it?

You did that.

You're still the same person that got that great night. And that means… you can do it again.

Yep, that's called a safety thought.

Making Life Tough for Insomnia

Many sleep therapists and doctors will tell you taking a nap is fine. After all, the people of the Mediterranean countries take a siesta every afternoon.

And taking a siesta *is* fine... if you're a Mediterranean without a sleep problem.

But then, drinking coffee at midnight, playing computer games in bed, lying in until noon are all fine activities... *if you don't have a sleep problem.*

Don't give your insomnia an easy opportunity to kick in. The boring name for avoiding naps, never reading in bed and sticking to a good routine is 'sleep hygiene'. But you can think of it as 'causing trouble for your insomnia'.

Don't give insomnia an easy ride.

Tired All Day No Matter What?

Patricia told me today that she is getting nothing but very, very light unrefreshing sleep. She can get 9, 10, 11 hours of sleep, and yet *still* feel exhausted all day. Many others have told me they seem to feel rough no matter how much sleep they get.

There can be many reasons for poor quality sleep, but before looking for other explanations, you really should go back to experimenting with Promise 1, *Spending Less Time in Bed*. I know it's the most boring promise, but it is also probably the most effective.

If you are spending 11 hours in bed *no wonder* you feel rough. If I spent 11 hours sleeping I would feel disastrous all day.

Spending far too *long* in bed seems to 'thin out' your sleep, decreasing its quality. Spending *less* time in bed often has the effect of 'squashing' the sleep into a more concentrated packet. For many of you, this will have the happy consequence of forcing you into deep delicious delta sleep.

And you will feel so much better.

Break the State

If you have been lying in bed for hours, tossing and turning, you know the best thing to do is get out of bed. But don't use this time out of bed just to lie on the sofa relaxing. This will do nothing to change your anxious state of mind.

The idea behind getting out of bed when you can't sleep is *not* to stay drowsy, or to 'get sleepier' as fast as you can. This will just continue the focus on the fact you aren't sleeping and worsen the worry.

Remember, you get out of bed to break *out* of that anxious state, not stay in in it. So do something completely different. Have a shower, walk the dog, clean the oven, draw a picture. One of my clients, Tessa, tells me she gets a big pile of ironing ready, just in case she needs to get out of bed!

In other words, do *anything* not concerned with sleep!

Thinking Is More Important Than Doing

One of the commonest mistakes people make in following my Method is in focussing on the first six promises - the basic sleep hygiene rules.

The truth is, these first six promises are really less than half the story. My method really only works so well because of the second six promises – those that address the negative thoughts and beliefs that always accompany and reinforce a chronic insomnia problem.

In fact, if you could get the thinking right, there would be almost no need for sleep hygiene at all.

I Prescribe a Course of Chilling Out

Do you often lie down with a pounding heart and a tight jaw? Are you waking up after only a few hours, or with stiff, aching joints? If so, you need to address your tension levels.

So many people leave this bit out.

We all know we *ought* to be putting aside time to de-stress, exercise or chill out. But there never seem to be enough hours in the day. So anxiety-reducing activities get pushed to the bottom of the 'to do' pile...and forgotten. But if you're a tense, anxious person, your sleeping patterns will not improve dramatically until you make relaxation a priority. You see, when you are really, really tense, it doesn't much matter whether you avoid reading, avoid naps, spend this or that time in bed, use this or that technique or even if you resort to sleeping aids and pills...if you are still very tense and anxious when it comes to bedtime, very often *nothing* will make you sleep.

I've said it before and I'll doubtless say it again...de-stressing is not optional, it is *prescribed.*

Yoga, meditation, reflexology, cycling, walking, Zumba classes, massage, aromatherapy... de-stressing can actually be *fun.*

Must You Give Up the Drugs First?

I am often asked whether it's necessary to come off all medication *before* starting *The Effortless Sleep Method*. This is a very common question. Some of you worry that taking sleeping medication will affect the working of the promises. Others are too scared even to start until they have completely kicked all the pills.

Let me assure you: there is no need to give up medication completely before starting on the method. In fact, the promises will only make it easier for you to give up. One of the reasons giving up medication is so hard is that you have nothing with which to replace it. The safety net is gone and in its place is often rebound insomnia.

One of my readers, Gracie, recently told me that following my method helped enormously in her attempt to give up her eight year sleeping pill habit, by teaching her to sleep naturally *as* she cut down. This method can go some way to taking the place of those pills. It can be your new safety net, just as it was hers.

So your faith and confidence in your *own ability to sleep* is *slowly* rediscovered, re-ignited and reborn.

So don't wait. Start the Method *and* your new life today

I Tell It Like It Is

I know I can be a bit bossy, a bit pushy. I don't sugar-coat the message and perhaps I sometimes don't sound particularly loving or caring.

But I do tell it like it is.

I tell it like it is because being sympathetic and loving isn't going to cure your insomnia.

And I'm not just here to help those who are already open to such ideas. I'm also here for those who are very sceptical. The truth is, I particularly want to help you 'tough nuts'. I particularly want this because I know what it is like to be you...

I know, because a 'tough nut' is exactly what I was for 15 years

The Fear Paradox

Is the unnecessary and exaggerated fear of missing one night enough to keep you awake?

If you can accept, really accept that you might not sleep, *and be ok with it* ... then fear *loses its grip.*

Paradoxical though it sounds, when you don't mind about missing sleep, you are more likely to get it!

A One Day Experiment

Just for one day, try to get through until bedtime without saying anything negative about your sleep, either to others or silently to yourself.

If this is difficult, impossible or you feel resistance even to the suggestion, then I know exactly where your problem lies.

When I say 'stop the negative sleep talk', this is not some airy-fairy, throwaway comment. Stopping negative sleep talk is *imperative* to success in overcoming insomnia.

Slow on the Uptake

If you are just starting out on your insomnia recovery, success can be erratic. Many people experience one or two good nights simply after reading the book. But this sudden positive reaction doesn't always last. When the initial 'glow' has worn off, it is often followed by a little run of poor sleep, and you can easily become despondent again.

But just think about this... if hope and positivity can give you even *one* good night, this should prove to you: this same positivity can give two, three nights and eventually a lifetime of good sleep.

Let me assure you, if you have *any* experience of sleeping better due to 'positive thinking', or from changing your thoughts, or feeling hope and then seeing a positive result in your sleep, *then you can become a brilliant, natural, effortless sleeper*.

That same mechanism which allowed thought to affect your sleep on one single night can be strengthened and honed to making you into a truly great sleeper.

Put It to the Test

If you don't believe you can change your beliefs about sleep at will, why not test the hypothesis? Pick another belief you don't currently have, preferably one that isn't too far from what you currently believe, create an affirmation for the belief ... *and keep repeating it.*

Try to imagine life as if this new belief were true. Speak to people, and answer questions as if you already believed it.

I promise you: even after one day you will notice you are feeling slightly different. Keep it up and eventually you'll find the belief will change.

It's not magic, it's just how the mind works.

It's Good to Be Ordinary

Because insomnia can feel so lonely, and so much like no one understands what you are going through, and because sleeping pills and other remedies haven't helped, it's hardly surprising that you begin to believe that there is something different, something unusual, something more severe about your insomnia.

Did you not realise that *every* insomniac believes this at some point or another?

There are 60 million people in the UK alone and between 10-30% are suffering with insomnia. Almost all of them believe their insomnia is different.

Just think about it … this would mean there are at least 6 million different types of insomnia, just in this one little country. How likely is that?

Just for once, it's great to be ordinary.

We All Do It

If you 'make a mistake', by succumbing to a sleeping pill, or lying in too late in the morning, don't beat yourself up and fall into negativity.

Remember, the commitment to being positive about your sleep is just as important …no, it is *more* important than bedtime habits or avoiding sleeping pills. Just get back on the horse and relax in the knowledge that *everyone* makes mistakes on this programme.

Focus on the End Result

Keep the end in sight, keep the end in sight, keep the end in sight!

If you are trying to walk to a destination in the far distance, you don't stop every time you stumble over a stone. You don't focus on the stone, worry about the stone, and say "Now, why did *that* happen? What did I do wrong?" No, you pay no attention to the stone, refocus on where you are headed, and keep going.

So why do you fall to bits every time you have a similar trip-up with sleep? Why do you focus on that one bad night, rather than on where you are going? Why worry about the one bad night rather than all the good ones waiting for you in the distance?

I don't know how close you are to the goal of perfect sleep, but I know the fastest way to get there is not to stop.

Overcoming Your Number One Issue

Hey you know that thing? You know: the thing your insomnia is all about? If *only* you could beat, learn to deal with, or get over that 'thing', you could *sleep!* If only you could find the right therapist, or technique, or pill which would get you over that thing, you would be cured. Right?

Wrong!

The truth is, that 'thing' is just something you mind has latched onto to try to make sense of all this. So when that 'thing' finally gets sorted, there will be another dozen 'things' all waiting in line to be the next 'thing' that your insomnia is all about.

Because that 'thing' is almost *never* what your insomnia is all about!

How to Get It Right

One of the most common questions I am asked by my therapy clients is 'am I getting it right?'

'How many hours, exactly, should I spend in bed?', 'how many times per week should I exercise?', 'is my safety thought correct?', 'is Pilates a good relaxation method, or should I do yoga instead?' Should I do this, that or the other?

If you constantly wonder and worry whether you are 'getting it right' or whether you are doing all the correct things to make the perfect sleep conditions, then you are *not getting it right!*

There is taking advice, and there is religiously obsessing over the details of that advice. There is sticking to the programme, and there is being constantly preoccupied with the programme. The promises of The Effortless Sleep Method are not hard-and-fast *rules.* Keep to them, but don't become obsessed with them.

Sleep is something you *let* happen, not *make* happen. Conditions should be conducive, but in fussing over making them perfect, you ensure they remain far from being so.

You are not going to cure insomnia by finding the ideal, perfect, magical time at which to go to bed, or the perfect amount of exercise or the perfect level of any other very specific action.

When you obsess about getting it right, if you don't sleep one night, you'll conclude you did something wrong. You'll imagine it's because you went to bed at the wrong time, or because you didn't exercise enough. And so you'll change things. And then if you still don't sleep, you'll change things again. And this frantic search for the ideal sleep conditions will carry on and on.

So, if you want to get it right, *don't fuss too much about getting it right.*

Why Do I Repeat Myself So Much?

When reading this book, it may seem that many of my stories repeat the same subjects. Sleeping pills, early waking, fear of missing sleep… Why do I need to repeat myself so often? Have I run out of things to say?

Not exactly!

If you look closely you'll see that while the same subjects may crop up time and time again, I cover them in a quite different way each time, addressing different aspects, different solutions and different ways of seeing the same situation.

And the truth is, some of these more important topics warrant an entire *book* of advice on their own.

But until those important books are written, a few extra stories should keep you going.

It's a Matter of Identity

Start becoming aware of the way *you* may be identifying yourself as 'an insomniac'.

We are striving for a time when you no longer see yourself as having a problem. All of the promises I ask you to make are designed to create a new identity for yourself as a 'Good Sleeper'.

While you still identify with your problem, consider yourself an insomniac, and talk and act from this place, nothing will really ever change, no matter what you do.

But if you could lose this insomniac identity, the problem would disappear of its own accord, without the need for any special steps, promises or even sleep hygiene.

The Not-So-Serious Rules
of The Good Sleepers' Club

The first rule of the Good Sleepers' Club is

Don't talk about insomnia

The second rule of the Good Sleepers' Club is

Don't talk about insomnia

Good Sleepers don't even have the word 'insomnia' in their vocabulary.

The Very Serious Rules of
The Good Sleepers' Club

1. *Expect the best*, assume that your sleep will become brilliant, perfect.

2. *Let everything be okay* – never, ever negatively judge your sleep. See only the good, and deny all that could be judged as bad.

3. *Bring it on* – get on with your life without one single compromise to your sleep.

For Early Wakers

This is for any newcomers who are suffering with sleep maintenance insomnia. Sleep maintenance insomniacs can usually fall asleep quite easily; their problem is with *staying* asleep. They will often wake in the early morning, after as little as two hours, and find they are unable to get back to sleep.

Sleep Maintenance Insomnia is *almost* always a sign of a general background tension and often appears when a person is experiencing a *particular* stress in their lives. Sleep maintenance insomnia can even pop up for really great sleepers when they are under extreme stress. (It has even happened to me occasionally for short periods.)

When this happens, your body is really just looking after you. It is allowing you just enough sleep to survive, and then waking you to deal with the terrible danger it thinks is imminent.

Now, it may be that this type of insomnia will disappear all on its own once the stressor has been removed. But you can also destabilise this kind of insomnia at its foundations by taking action to remove tension and deal with the physical and emotional stress.

By taking direct action to tackle tension and stress levels *throughout the day*, a person can often cure themselves almost instantly of this problem. Deal with the stress and your body will stop 'stopping' you from sleeping.

This will also have the additional benefit of making you feel better and be better able to deal with the difficult circumstance which may have caused the stress in the first place.

But don't leave it until you go to bed to relax. Work on tension levels during the day, and there'll be no need to do much at bedtime. You could see this early waking magically disappear simply by introducing a regular de-stressing activity into your life. Meditation, massage, yoga, dancing, watching comedy or simply vigorous exercise can work wonders with this type of issue. I leave the choice of activity to you.

Why Am I So Down on Sleeping Pills?

In *The Effortless Sleep Method* I described in detail the many negative side-effects of sleeping medications.

Now, hear this … sleeping pills do *not* even make you sleep. That's right; they do *not* make you sleep. What they *do* is one of two things:

1. They knock you unconscious – not causing real, natural normal sleep, but drugged unconsciousness. There is *always* a high degree of hangover in this case, as the amount of genuine sleep obtained is minimal.

2. They give you faith and trust, which relaxes you enough to actually fall sleep – in effect, acting in a somewhat similar way to placebo. This is why some find a tiny crumb of pill effective. Similarly, those people finding themselves awake in the early hours, and who are able to fall asleep *within seconds* of taking a pill, are also relying on little other than placebo.

In this case, the pill does have an effect, just not the intended one. The effect it has is a negative one – making you feel groggy and possibly anxious the next day.

I'm not down on pills because of some New Age self-righteous idea about 'naturalness' and avoiding 'drugs' because they are inherently 'bad' or sinful in some way.

I say this because medications, both prescribed and over-the-counter, *do not cure insomnia.*

The aim of this programme is to rediscover and rekindle your own, natural ability to sleep. The taking of sleeping pills is in direct opposition to this approach. If you take a sleeping pill every night, you should speak to your doctor about reducing the dosage with a view to giving up altogether.

Just Do Nothing...

So many people worry about what to *do* when they get into bed. And, once they have decided on what to 'do' (for example, a relaxation method), they then worry about whether they are doing it properly.

For this reason, I really recommend that everyone experiments with the 'doing nothing' technique I talk about in *The Effortless Sleep Method*. After all, this is what every normal sleeper 'does' every night. And, it may surprise you to know (it surprised me) that more of *you* report success with this technique than any other I recommend.

Try it tonight. Just go to bed and *do* absolutely nothing. If thoughts arise, don't stop them. If you want to move, move. If your heart pounds, let it. If emotion or fear arise, don't resist. Just let it all *be.*

And...if you find yourself getting sleepier and dropping off, don't try and hold onto that sleepy feeling or try and replicate what you think you were doing to make that happen. Just continue to *do* nothing at all.

You may just surprise yourself...

All That Matters Is How You Feel

Claire tells me there is something wrong with her because she can't nap; Jakob worries that he always takes an hour to fall asleep; Melissa is concerned that she always has to wake up and use the toilet at night.

Imagining that everyone else in the world doesn't *also* experience these things, well that's just plain nonsense. I know countless *non*-insomniac people who are never able to nap, take an hour to fall asleep and who almost never sleep through the night. (I am one of them.)

These things are not a problem for people like us because we don't see them as problems. In fact, we don't even think about them. The sleep we do get is deep and delicious, we have tons of energy and we generally feel good all day.

But, if we fussed and fretted about *why* we can't do what others find so easy then we would be in trouble too.

Don't judge your sleep according to external norms. All that matters is how well you feel, no matter how long or how broken your sleep.

Give Yourself Some Credit

As I have said many times before. I cannot *make* you sleep. What I *can* do is to show you how to change your thoughts and behaviours. I can show you how to create the optimum physical and psychological conditions for good sleep to occur. It's up to you to put all that into practice.

Next time you get a good night's sleep, remember: that's not something I have done. So don't give me the credit. *You* did that. *You* got a good night's sleep, on your own.

So give yourself credit where credit's due.

In fact, 'big yourself up' about it, bask in it, revel in it. You got a good night's sleep, and that's just brilliant

*

Meditate Your Way to Sleep

If you are serious about changing your life for the better you should think about starting a daily meditation practice.

Don't dismiss this as the usual generic 'you just need to relax' advice. Daily meditation can have an astonishing, almost immediate effect on anxiety levels. Take up daily meditation and any anxiety could become a thing of the past. 'Deep-seated issues' will bother you less, and you may find new insights regarding them. The most common effect of meditation is that people report 'not being bothered about things so much'. Life just becomes subtly easier and easier, freer and lighter.

Meditation alone may not cure chronic insomnia, but it will make all the other steps much more effective.

My Absolute Favourite Insomnia-Killing Relaxation Regime

The following is a wonderful practice which will make a profound difference to your sleep and your life in general. Meditate *twice* a day using a mantra or watching the breath, for 20 to 30 minutes, morning and early evening. Twice a day works *far* better than just once and has way more than double the effect of a single meditation!

Then, at bedtime, meditate sitting in bed in the darkness for just a few minutes until you feel yourself starting to nod off. Gently lie down, paying no attention to anything in particular. Just lie there, do nothing and let your thoughts drift.

Many of you have reported that this practice will often allow you to fall asleep almost instantly. And it was after doing this that I had my first ever experience of 'being asleep before my head hit the pillow.'

Putting Your Mind to Bed

Do you have a troublesome issue which is occupying your thoughts at night, going around and around, and making sleep difficult? Or do you find yourself always replaying the day's events in your mind, just before bed?

Instead of trying to block or stop these thoughts, sometimes it can help to do the following:

Allocate yourself 15 or 20 minutes before bed, during which you are allowed to think about your issues; think whatever you like, come up with a solution, or just let the thoughts swirl around. For 20 minutes, it's 'thinking time' and your mind can do what it likes.

Then, when the time is up, just tell yourself thinking time is over until tomorrow night, and move your mind to another subject.

Sometimes, this little bit of time is all your mind is craving. Give it free rein for 20 minutes and quite often it will then shut up for the rest of the night.

Putting Your Mind on Paper

I spoke recently of a method for dealing with troublesome thoughts at bedtime – by allowing yourself a set amount of time to indulge them, letting them play out, and then moving on.

Another method which you may find extremely helpful is to always have a pencil and paper next to the bed. If you are struck by a sudden thought, remember something you should have done today, or should do tomorrow, or even have a new insight or idea, do the following:

Turn on the light and write down a note to yourself.

Tell yourself : *I can't do anything about the issue now. But come tomorrow, this note will remind me to deal with it appropriately.*

By getting the thoughts out of your head and down onto paper, they will no longer persist in nagging at you. This will allow you to 'put the issue to bed' for now, safe in the knowledge that you will take care of everything properly in the morning.

Simple, but effective.

It Happens to All of Us

If you miss a night, please don't automatically assume that your 'insomnia is back'. If you cannot accept the odd bad night you will remain trapped in a pattern of catastrophising after every 'less than perfect' night.

You need to understand that one bad night is not something that non-insomniacs fear at all, even though it happens to them more often than you might realise.

Everyone, and I mean *everyone*, has a bad night from time to time.

When You've Done Everything
in Your Power

Michael wrote a while ago to tell me there must be something really wrong with him. He explained to me that he was taking a combination of prescribed and over-the-counter medication plus alcohol, using a special 'earthing sheet' on the bed, a hypnosis CD, special acupressure jewellery, eye-shades and ear-plugs and *still* he could not sleep.

Poor Michael didn't realise just how 'normal' he really was. It was all his extra paraphernalia which was abnormal.

I told him, the more sleep aids he uses, the more elaborate the routine, the more he attends to 'making himself sleep', the lesser his chances of sleeping.

Michael wrote again yesterday. He's now sleeping much better, taking nothing to bed but a pair of underpants!

Not Understanding *AGAIN*

Why do I keep banging on about understanding this, seeing that, realising the other? Why don't I just tell you how to jolly well sleep?!

Because... it's only by understanding this, seeing that and realising the other, that you will truly learn to jolly well sleep!

Understanding is everything

I Can't Do Magic

It's very common that people read my books, and then sleep really well for a couple of nights just on the strength of the hope they afford. But this happy outcome can be misleading and can overshadow a hidden danger.

After this initial success, some people assume they are then cured. Job done! As if overcoming insomnia happens by simply reading the words. But when an inevitable bad night comes along, they wonder what has gone wrong. I get so many people write to me to tell me the method has suddenly stopped working, after two or three *days*. Presumably they think that the act of reading a book is going to cure their insomnia.

It reminds me of an ancient Chinese proverb which reads:

"To know and not do is not to know."

Following my method means following my method. It does not mean reading the book, getting all psyched up and then sitting back and waiting for things to happen. Nor is it enough to follow the easier bits of sleep hygiene and leave out all the bits that take a bit more effort. The method works, but it isn't magic. You can't just read the words and the spell is cast. You have to follow the instructions too!

Plan in Advance

Got a new technique or relaxation method to try? If so, *please* don't make the mistake of waiting until a high-pressure night, comes along to try it - before the weddings, the important meetings, the job interviews…

This is a mistake most insomniacs make again and again.

If you wait until a really high-pressure night, the unfamiliarity of any new technique, added to the stress of the situation will mean there is almost no chance your sleeping. This will then add to your despondency and the feeling of 'nothing ever working'.

Let anything new become familiar before you deem it a failure.

Look to the End Result

Did you know... a show-jumper always focuses attention on the ground after the jump? If he or she focuses on the jump itself, the horse will crash or refuse.

Similarly, a martial artist never focuses on the point of impact when striking an opponent, but rather on the space beyond that point.

Don't focus on tonight. Don't focus on what you will or will not do in order to precipitate good sleep. Instead, turn your focus to tomorrow. Focus on feeling good, waking up refreshed, going about your day feeling bright and happy. Focus on this enough, and your mind find a way to make it real...

Master focusing on the next day, and the night will take care of itself.

I Am an Ex-Insomniac...

Have you noticed the way that ex-smokers get a real kick out of saying 'I don't smoke'? Have you also noticed that they often begin affirming their new non-smoking status just *days* after having given up?

They are already living the new non-smoking lifestyle, trying it on for size, creating a new identity, before the cravings have even stopped. It can be the same with your sleep...

You don't have to wait until it's true to start boasting!

Have You Been Researching
Sleep Forums Again?

Have you scared yourself witless by reading insomnia horror stories online? Have you been reading that it can take *years* to fully give up sleeping medication? Have you read that some people *never* recover? Are you now anticipating another 30 years of insomnia?

Remember, when it comes to insomnia forums:

1. There is absolutely no reason to believe that your recovery or experience will be anything like the experiences of those few you read online.

2. People who post on forums tend to be those with very bad experiences. All the millions that manage to give up medication, and overcome insomnia with relatively little trouble *almost never bother to post online about it.*

I'm Tired, Just Tired, That's All

I didn't get much sleep last night. Yep, that's right, I didn't sleep. I was up all night dealing with a case of copyright infringement. An old therapy client of mine has taken my material and used it to create a string of Youtube videos and a Facebook page. By the time I finished working it was getting light. I lay in bed for another hour, creating stories and conversations in my head, thinking of things I should or shouldn't do or say. There was no way I was going to sleep. So I got up.

I have had a fully sleepless night....

So why am I telling you this? It's because once again, I am struck by how much better a lack of sleep feels *when it's not a case of insomnia,* when I am not adding anxiety to the feeling of sleep deprivation. I'm tired...no, I'm *exhausted.* But there is no stressing about it, no panic, no tears, no 'it's all gone wrong!' I have had a good breakfast, a great cup of coffee and I'm getting on with my day. I expect by evening I will be feeling almost normal. Now, if it's this easy to deal with non-insomnia sleeplessness, we ought to be able to cope equally well with insomnia-based sleeplessness.

If you could only get a sense of this for yourself, it could really turn things around.

Silly Triggers

In the early days of recovery, little seemingly insignificant things can suddenly begin affecting your sleep. Examples might be a partner staying over, a partner staying away, having sex before sleep, or even a particular day of the week.

Often this can be the exact opposite of what used to be true for you. For example, you might find that the hour of TV, the half hour of reading, the hot drink, the chat in bed which once settled you down nicely, has suddenly started to disturb you.

When you *know* there is no sense to these reactions, the worst thing you can do is to avoid the triggers. Don't keep your partner from staying, or give up your nightly reading. Avoidance just marks these things out as special, as danger. They then take on inflated significance until they become a perfect, absolute, reliable trigger for a bad night.

Read your books, enjoy your bedtime cuddle, have your partner stay every day for *weeks*, until that silly habit breaks.

Acceptance not Stagnation

Many people become frustrated when they hear me give the following advice.

"You need to learn to stop caring about missing sleep."

This makes some people very angry. It makes them angry because they think this sort of acceptance means learning to live with insomnia, learning to put up with insomnia, resigning themselves to it.

It doesn't. Acceptance doesn't mean stagnation at all. Learning to be ok with your current problem means your current problem will begin to improve.

Strange, I know. But I promise, it's true

Why Wait?

What does lack of sleep stop you from doing? Are you looking forward to a time when your sleep is good enough to allow you to do those things...all those things you have put off because you have insomnia?

If only you realised: by 'putting things off because of insomnia', you only reinforce that insomnia.

The truth is, really good reliable sleep will only come *after* you start doing those things, not before.

So why not do one of those things today?

What Makes You Think
It's Purely Physical?

I get *so* many people write to me to tell me they can't, or won't follow certain pieces of my advice because they firmly believe there is a medical or physical reason for their insomnia.

In my experience, insomniacs are notoriously *bad* at knowing what is best when it comes to their problem. They are also prone to over-diagnosis and obsessing about treatments.

Now, I'm not saying there can never be a physical reason behind your insomnia. What I am saying is that there is probably no way for you to tell how much (if any) of the insomnia is down to the physical affliction, and how much (if any) of it is simply down to your behaviours, thoughts and beliefs about sleep.

So, why not just follow the advice anyway?

We've All Been There

If you are in a bad place right now, perhaps desperate, panicking, sinking into the abyss, can't take any more...then you may find some comfort in this thought.

Every person who has ever overcome insomnia using this method (and there have been tens of thousands now) has been exactly where you are now. Every good sleeper was once a really bad sleeper, just like you. Every one of us has felt desperate, panicky, on the brink of utter despair. We have all wondered the same things: 'Am I different, why am I not responding properly, am I doing something wrong, why isn't it working, why has it all gone wrong again?'

We have all thought all of these things, and we have all come through it to a better place, to a life of normal, blissful sleep.

No Wonder You Can't Sleep

If you are under unusually high levels of stress at the moment, don't make the mistake of thinking that an inability to sleep is an indication of serious insomnia. Remember, an inability to sleep is also your body's normal, natural response to stress. It is simply trying to keep you safe by making sure you are alert enough to deal with the danger at hand.

In such circumstances, it is helpful if you can stop concentrating on the sleep itself. Instead, find a way to relax and de-stress *in preparation* for sleep so that it is easier to sleep when you finally lie down. Use exercise, yoga, meditation or your own favourite method.

It may be that your sleep will not go completely back to normal until your life becomes a little less difficult.

Try not to add worry about insomnia to your already hectic life

Special Events – Forgetting to Remember

One of the most difficult things to cope with is what I call 'special event insomnia' - the infuriating tendency to sleep really badly before the most important, fun or 'special' events.

The reason you cannot sleep before important or exciting events is simply down to the heightened state of excitement and expectation that occurs when you are looking forward to, or are apprehensive about, a future event.

The normal good sleeper is not disturbed by this kind of thing, but your sleep may not yet be strong enough to allow this.

But it will change.

If you're just starting out, try not to worry too much about these nights. If you are anything like me, this 'sleeping before events' will be the last part of your problem to disappear.

Focus on improving your sleep on all those 'normal' nights first. In the beginning, the tiniest thing can trigger a bad night, perhaps an early start, or having to make a particular phone call in the morning.

But as your sleep begins to improve, you'll find that the nights you classify as 'special' or 'high-pressure' will naturally begin to change. And you will find yourself sleeping before bigger and more important days.

And finally, one morning, you will find yourself having slept really well before an event which would once have terrified you. And then, the thought will hit you... *I forgot to worry about sleep.*

What You Focus on...

I'm fond of saying *whatever you focus on gets bigger.*

Now, what do you suppose happens when you *obsess* about something, night and day?

That's right; it gets so big it takes over your entire life.

So, what do you think would happen if you only ever obsessed about the *good* nights?

Keep thinking…

Nothing Can Make You Sleep

Do you approach sleep aids and techniques as if they were a 'cure' that can *make* you sleep? Do you lie in bed, waiting for them to work?

The fact is, no method or technique has the power to *make* you sleep. Sleeping is not something that any external thing can 'do' to you. Nothing can *make* you sleep, not my method as laid out in the book, not even sleeping pills (although they can force you into unconsciousness). Sleeping is something that will happen naturally and *automatically* when all the circumstances are right. Sleeping is something you *allow* to happen, not something you make happen.

All that I can do for you is to help make sure those circumstances are as favourable as possible.

It's Not Insomnia

Insomniacs tend to forget that such things as noise, funny sleeping hours or a strange bed will disturb even a great sleeper.

If you don't sleep in a hotel bed, or while neighbours are having an all-night party this shouldn't immediately signal insomnia.

There's no way to determine whether this sort of sleeplessness is 'insomnia', or is just a perfectly normal reaction to a disturbance.

Try not to be *overly* concerned about those nights. They can be very misleading. So when considering your own progress, remember to throw these nights out of the equation.

How Do I Maintain the Good Sleep?

So, you are in a good spell. How do you ensure that this spell continues?

What you must 'do' now is *do nothing*.

Begin to let go, let go of the worrying, the wondering. When things are going well, it's easy to become obsessed with trying to make sure the good sleep continues.

Recognise that you are truly, absolutely, genuinely getting better and leave it at that. Just relax and realise the enormity of what you have just achieved. Smile and bask in the gorgeousness of good sleep.

Many people go 30 years without your sort of success, believe it!

How to Look Forward to Big Events

'Special event insomnia' really can be tedious. This is the miserable experience of being totally unable to sleep before important events. This problem can take a long time to get over and sometimes lingers long after the rest of your sleep has become excellent. I get asked a lot about this issue and I really want to help you all nail it.

If you are already plagued by fearful thoughts of an upcoming event, try a little technique that I have been telling my therapy clients about. Maria told me just this morning that this technique allowed her to sleep well on the night before her sister's wedding, an event she had worried over for months:

Quieten your mind for a few minutes. And then, imagine yourself going to bed on this 'special' night. Imagine yourself feeling so tired and sleepy that you collapse into your comfy bed, heavy and grateful. The tiredness is so overwhelming that it envelops you instantly, and you fall into a delicious sleep, deep as the ocean. Don't just visualise, really *feel* it in your body.

Then do it again.

The first few times you try to imagine this, it may not work. Your mind may try and jump in to sabotage things. But persevere; it will become easier. The idea is to replace those habitual fearful thoughts with more positive ones. Eventually, your mind will become used to this thought, and the imagining will become easy, automatic.

Then, when you are going about your everyday life and a fearful thought of that future event pops into your mind, immediately replace it with that lovely thought of collapsing into bed, overcome with sleepiness. Do this enough, and you won't even have to try anymore; the lovely relaxing thought will pop in automatically. You have created an association between a special night, and the deepest, most delicious sleep ever.

The very least this will do is to neutralise that everyday niggling fear of the upcoming event. But do it enough, and the fear will have disappeared so much that you will find yourself sleeping, before *any* event.

Dealing with Bad Nights

There *will* be more bad nights, I promise you.

The determining factor in whether you turn out to be a success or a failure in the fight against insomnia, will not just concern the *good* nights.

It will be largely about how you deal with those *bad* nights.

Will you panic, stress out and 'wonder what you did wrong'? …

Or accept them, ignore them, and keep looking forward to the next bit of good sleep?

Poor Old You

You will find it harder to cope, and much harder to be positive, on those days when you feel rotten. But don't make the mistake of beating yourself up for not coping, or not feeling positive. If you have missed 2, 3 or more days, and you are feeling like death, stop fighting it. The worst thing you can do is to beat yourself up for feeling bad or panicking.

Just allow yourself to feel like rubbish. Allow it, really allow it, and it will begin to pass, or at least start feeling a little lighter.

A positive thought can just be: 'I feel terrible today, so I'm going to be extra kind to myself. Tomorrow will be a better day'. As long as the general 'thrust' of your thoughts is in a positive direction, they will increase.

Sometimes, just being kind to yourself is positivity enough

Obsession I

I admit it: I'm a total obsessive. I have an unbelievably obsessive personality. But I don't ever seek to do anything about this character trait. I certainly don't want some therapist to 'fix' it.

When obsession is about useless, destructive things, like finding an external cure for something which can only be cured by looking within, or with trying to work out 'why me?' then obsession becomes desperate, crazy even.

But an obsessive personality can also be a real asset – it helps you to get projects finished, find inspired new ways of doing things, and allows you to think and think and think until some real insight occurs.

So rejoice in your obsessive personality, but put it to good use.

Obsession II

I can't just tell you to 'stop obsessing' about sleep. That's just like asking you not to think of a white bear. You'll only end up obsessing about how to stop obsessing about sleep!

If you're an obsessive type, the answer is to find a *new* obsession, – *one which enriches your life*. If strong enough, it will very effectively redirect your attention – to the extent that you actually forget about your sleep problems.

Because no one has room for more than one fully-fledged obsession.

A 60 Day Commitment

It is going to take more than a few nights or weeks of good sleep to permanently overcome chronic insomnia. You need to keep up the good habits until they become ingrained, become automatic, become 'the norm'.

Apparently, it takes 60 days to create a 'permanent' habit. So make the commitment to giving it *at least* this long.

If Only There Were A Pill...

Perhaps there *is* a pill which will cure your insomnia – one you just haven't tried yet?

Just a few nights of good sleep might just set you on the right path, and get some stability back into your life…

…if only.

The lie told about sleeping pills is that they are prescribed to those with short term insomnia in order to normalise sleeping patterns.

The truth is somewhat different. 65% of sleeping pills currently taken are being prescribed to those who have been taking them for an average of *five years*.

So *please* think twice before deciding a new pill is the answer

It Is Gone, Never to Return

Do you know how I can *know* that insomnia will never come back for me?

It's because I no longer care whether or not I will sleep.

If I miss a night, I pay no attention to it. Even if I missed two, three nights (which never happens any more), I wouldn't be happy about it, but it wouldn't signal insomnia for me. I wouldn't panic. I would just get on with life and look forward to sleeping again. Insomnia will never have me in its grasp again because I'm just not scared of it any more.

If you can learn to think this way too, one bad night will almost inevitably turn out to be just *one* bad night.

Whatever's Good for You

A really good night of quality sleep would probably be made up of the optimum amounts of each of the various sleep stages - light sleep, REM sleep and deep Delta sleep.

However, I think it's important not to quantify this in any kind of objective way. For a start, it's almost impossible to know these things accurately without having an expensive sleep study.

There is no point getting into a panic over whether you are getting this or that amount of this or that type of sleep. It is this sort of attention to detail which leads people to think there is something wrong with them if they get less than eight hours.

Good quality sleep is that which means you are able to get out of bed without *too* much difficulty, and have a full and productive day, through until bedtime without exhaustion sullying things for you.

In short, if you feel you are getting quality sleep, then you probably are. If lack of sleep is negatively affecting your life, you will know it, and you won't need an external yardstick to tell you this.

Only Keep the Best Bits

I once thought that incessant worry, depression, negative thinking and insomnia were just part of who I was. There was no point in trying to change these things.

Moreover, why *should* I change if these things were part of my very *character?*

These days, I just don't allow any of that rubbish into my head any more. I'm still obsessive and over-analytical, but now I'm happy almost all the time.

And who knows, perhaps I'll no longer be obsessive and over-analytical when I stop telling that particular story.

Dying of Insomnia?

About once or twice a month, someone contacts me convinced they have sporadic fatal insomnia. This is a type of severe insomnia which actually results in death. This prospect is terrifying for the fledgling insomniac and perhaps most of us have worried, at some point, that we might have this horrible condition.

Let's get things in perspective for a moment: somewhere between 10-30% of the world's population suffers with insomnia. That's at least 7,000,000,000 insomniacs.

24,000 get struck by lightning every year. Around 100 people are attacked by sharks every year. There are around 1-2000 cases of bubonic plague every year.

There have only been *eight* recorded cases of sporadic fatal insomnia *ever*.

Eight.

There are more important things to worry about than sporadic fatal insomnia

Being a Good Friend

Most of you know by now that complaining about your sleep is not a good idea. But what do you do if friends or family begin to complain to you about *their* sleep?

First of all, this situation doesn't help you at all. Listening to the sleep worries of others can scare you and focus your attention back onto your own problem.

But besides this, it doesn't help *them* to have a willing listener for their gripes and worries. Give them advice if it's appropriate. But if you really want to be a good friend, *don't* indulge their complaints, their moans and their horror stories about sleep.

Things to Do During a Bad Patch

It's a shame that most people wait until a really bad patch of sleep to take action. Usually, they will wait until they are completely desperate and then begin trying things, scouring the internet for tips, listening to new CDs, putting in place lots of extra routines to do in bed.

But a really bad patch of sleep is the very worst time to begin something different. All this does is draw attention to the problem, mark the night out as different, and puts you in an even more conscious and alert state when actually going to bed.

The best thing you can do when in the middle of a really bad patch is *nothing special*. Do nothing 'different', nothing 'new'. Just keep the sleep hygiene good, keep your thoughts as positive as you can, accept that things are going to be difficult for a bit... and then just sit tight and wait for the next little run of good sleep. The more you can take your focus away from what is wrong, and towards a more accepting place, the better state you will be in for sleeping.

Building up Mental Strength

I came across this little quotation yesterday and it seemed to sum up perfectly the process of belief change through positive thinking, affirmations and slowly building on good experiences.

"Mental strength is secured in exactly the same way that physical strength is secured, by exercise. We think something, perhaps with difficulty the first time; we think the same thing again, and it becomes easier this time; we think it again and again, it then becomes a mental habit. We continue to think the same thing. Finally, it becomes automatic; we can no longer help thinking this thing. We are now positive of what we think; there is no longer any doubt about it. We are sure, we know." (Charles Haanel)

It's difficult at first, especially when it feel like no progress is being made. But every single time you think that new positive thought, it gets a tiny bit easier.

Overnight Cures?

Any peddler of an instant insomnia cure, any website which claims to have you sleeping within minutes, anyone who tells you they can cure your insomnia *right now*, is being somewhat economical with the truth.

Do you know why instant miracle cures will never work? Do you know why chronic insomnia can't be cured overnight?

It's because *belief* doesn't change overnight. After weeks, months or years of negative thinking, it takes more than a few days of good sleep to break through to that positive new belief. And changing belief is the biggest part of overcoming medium to long-term insomnia.

Sooner or later, you really need to give up that search.

Making Visualisation Effective

When I'm sleeping in a strange bed, I like to use a little visualisation to get me off to sleep. My current favourite is that I have been lost in the woods, stumbling in the dark, exhausted until I come across a perfect little magical hut, and inside it is the safest, most comfortable bed in the world. And as I actually get into bed and lie down, I imagine myself lying down into this wonderful imaginary bed.

This visualisation is entirely personal to me. It is something *I* find incredibly delicious and soothing. This is important. Because by making it a really fun and enjoyable visualisation, I can do it just for its own sake. I do it for fun, because I like it. I don't do it 'because I can't sleep'. Helping me sleep is just a welcome side-effect of this technique.

If you decide to try a visualisation, don't think you have to use a stock guided meditation from a CD or a download. It will work far better for sleep if you use one which is personal to *you*, one you would do just because you enjoy the experience.

(And if you do experiment with visualisation, and your mind starts to wander to something completely unrelated, *let it.)*

Affirmations for the Bad Days

When you feel like death through lack of sleep, affirming 'I'm the best sleeper in the world' probably isn't the best idea. It's all too easy for your mind to jump in and sabotage all your good intentions.

When you feel like this, pick a thought, any positive thought, which makes you feel a *little* calmer, a *little* clearer, a *little* more 'on track' and use that as the basis for your affirmation.

You could even affirm *I feel a little calmer, I feel a little clearer, I'm still on track and I'm getting better.*

Then resolve to have the best day you possibly can

Save 'I'm the best sleeper in the world' for those days when you sleep well!

'Doing Nothing' – With Bells On

This year I attended a weekend conference. Beforehand, I was actually looking forward to the prospect of a hotel stay – crisp white cotton sheets, free miniature shower gel and shampoo, fluffy towels all laid out for me....

Sadly, it turned out that my immediate neighbours (who were also at the conference) apparently didn't require sleep. At 2am they were still partying in their room, about six of them. What's more, they were smoking (illegal in UK hotels) and the smoke was coming through the vents into my room. It took three calls to reception and a large Polish security guard, threatening them with ejection from the hotel, to get them finally to be quiet. By this time, it was about 4am (I didn't actually look at the clock!) and I was furious. I needed to be up at 7.30 and was now in the worst possible state for sleeping. I was wound up, tense, and my mind was racing with angry thoughts. Here was I, a so-called sleep expert, wide awake in the middle of the night.

So…what to do?

Well, I realised that it was probably too late to get much of a sleep in now. It would take me far too long to calm down enough. So I just decided to lay on the bed and *rest*. I wouldn't do anything at all to make me sleep, I wouldn't do a relaxation, or an affirmation, or a bit of Sedona method… I would just *rest*. The room was now silent and peaceful. I would enjoy those crisp cotton sheets, that comfy bed and those soft pillows. I would just enjoy my surroundings and let tomorrow take care of itself. After all, it was really too late to do anything about it now.

Next thing I knew, my alarm was going off at 7.30. I hadn't even noticed myself relaxing, let alone getting sleepy. And yet I had had good deep sleep, albeit for only a few hours. And I really felt pretty good after a shower and a coffee. I can only put this success down to my total lack of *doing* anything 'to make me sleep'. All pressure to sleep was off and my mind and body just let go.

Can you work this idea of 'not doing' into your own difficult nights? Can you just all yourself to *rest*, to enjoy the wonderful luxury of your own comfy bed, for its own sake, without actually doing anything at all?

Try it...

Thanks to You Brian, for This Story

One of my readers sent me a lovely quotation. I don't usually just steal the words of others, but this was so beautiful and so apt.

"In the cellars of the night, when the mind starts moving around old trunks of bad times, the pain of this and the shame of that, the memory of a small boldness is a hand to hold." John Leonard, critic (1939 - 2008)

'A small boldness' – Like a poetic description of a safety thought.

Can You Sleep Fine, But Only in the Spare Room?

A lot of people worry that, although their sleeping has massively improved, they have come to use the spare room as a crutch and are now unable to sleep in their own bed. Perhaps your partner snores, or perhaps you worry about disturbing your partner!

Actually, don't think there is a huge problem with sleeping in the spare room, or even on the couch or sofa. The most important thing is that you are getting sleep. Full stop.

However, at some point you are going to want to change this. At some point you want to be sleeping normally, in your own bed.

But if it feels like a massive challenge to do this, then there is no need to rush things. Let yourself settle into a really good pattern of sleep even if that means sleeping in the spare room. When your confidence has improved dramatically, you will feel happy about going back to your own room. Take it easy, and celebrate every little success, no matter where that success takes place.

Is Insomnia Really a Life Sentence?

I'm aware that there are other insomnia writers out there who advise us to accept that insomnia tends to be a lifelong problem. Some are from the school of thought which says 'once an insomniac, always an insomniac'. Their answer is to learn to accept poor sleep, learn to live with it, and get on with life as best you can.

Rubbish.

First of all, this horribly self-fulfilling prophecy is totally disempowering. If you believe you'll probably never get better, you probably never will.

It also just *isn't true.*

I hear from people every day who having followed this simple advice, are now sleep better than they did before their insomnia began. People all over the world are reporting similar stories, some of them after suffering for 40 or even 50 years! One of my oldest readers is Bill, who at the age of 79, reports he now sleeping better than he can ever remember.

Leave the lifelong insomniacs to their negative views. You don't have to be part of their world, unless you choose to.

You Just Need One Good Night

The truth is, successful ex-insomniacs tend to have many, many setbacks. They still have nights where they don't sleep too well, and the old fear will return...

"Is my insomnia back?"

But successful people will always tend to cling on to one safety thought:

"If I slept well on ONE night, without drugs, without crutches, just on my own... then I can do it again."

And so can you

Life Is for Living... Now.

It can be very tempting to avoid all those things that could interfere with your sleep, including fun, important or special events. Is there a big event looming that you are too scared to attend? Are you worried that you might not sleep the night before? Are you even thinking of cancelling?

Please don't.

If you cancel, postpone or refuse to attend a big event, you pretty much guarantee the same thing will happen next time; this same worry will be present, and you will again think of cancelling. And this pattern will repeat, and repeat and repeat.

Go to your event and do your best to enjoy it. Because the only way to break this pattern, *is to break this pattern!* Just this move alone will start to weaken the negative habit, *even if you don't sleep*.

If you cancel important or fun events because you worry they could stop you from sleeping, you may avoid insomnia, *for one night..*

... but you will reinforce it *as a lifelong problem.*

When You Just Don't Have the Time

You all know how much I push the idea of a daily meditation practice. You've heard me talk about what an astonishingly positive effect it can have on sleep patterns and life in general.

So, I just thought I'd share this little quotation with you...

> "You should sit in meditation for 20 minutes a day,
> Unless you are too busy:
> Then you should sit for an hour."
> (Old Zen saying)

Too busy to exercise, meditate, or de-stress? Then you of all people need to exercise, meditate and de-stress.

It's Not Always Easy

Of *course* it is going to be harder to stay positive when you haven't slept well. Of course the affirmations are going to sound more like lies, of course it's going to be harder to 'put your life first' when exhaustion is clouding your thoughts. But *that's fine!*

Just do what you can, do your best – even one more gram, one more ounce, one more iota of positivity is better than none at all. Each and *every* time you think a positive thought, say an affirmation (and feel it), or reply with a positive answer, *your next good night comes a little closer!*

Sweet Memories

Think back to a time when you fell asleep really easily and deliciously. It may have been recently, or it may have been decades ago. For me, this 'effortless' sleep often happens on the train. The gentle movement lulls me so gently and persuasively, I can actually watch myself fall asleep.

Thomas, one of my therapy clients likes to recall a memory of falling asleep under a tree at Glastonbury festival, with the sound of distant music and murmuring voices. This happened many years ago for Thomas. But so lovely is the memory, that he now looks forward to bedtime so he can revisit his Glastonbury tree memory.

Next time you are lying in bed not sleeping, recall one of these times. Go back there. Gently float into that memory and feel those feelings of drifting, softly, deliciously into sleep. I have favourite memories like this that I call on again and again.

If you can't recall such a time, try making up an imaginary perfect sleep. (It works just as well!)

How to Have a Relapse

Do you know, I think I could quite easily have a 'relapse' (the dreaded word!) and go back to where I was? I could become a really terrible sleeper, completely obsessed with my problem again.

But what could cause this terrible turn of events?

If I focussed on the bad nights (which still very occasionally happen), the way I am feeling moment to moment, on the possibility that this, that or the other will affect my sleep, if I went back to researching, reading, talking about my problem. If I began testing every new medication and sleep aid on the market, if I stopped talking about how great my sleep is, if I looked to the negative instead of always, *always* to the positive, *I could go back there too!*

But don't be alarmed. Just make sure you do the opposite of all these things, and your chances of a serious relapse will be pretty much nil.

Antidepressants and Sleep

Have you been prescribed antidepressants for insomnia? We are often told that insomnia is a symptom of depression. But I am convinced it is usually the other way around.

Many people coming to me for help are taking antidepressants, even though most have never complained about depression to their doctor. Most of them are convinced that far from being caused *by* depression, insomnia has been *the cause* of their depression. Others say they never felt depressed *until they started taking the antidepressants*

If your antidepressants are working for you… great! I would never suggest you stop taking something which is genuinely helping.

But if you feel they are doing you no good, or are making things worse, be assured that this is a completely normal reaction. Don't imagine for one moment that a bad response to antidepressants means there is something extra 'wrong' with you.

Let's face it, if depression wasn't the cause of your insomnia in the first place, it's hardly surprising that an antidepressant doesn't cure it

I'm Getting Better, But...

Is your sleep improving, are negative thoughts decreasing, are you getting better...?

But the odd bad night or anxious thought still keeps popping up at inopportune times to scare you?

 Then focus on this: your sleep is improving, negative thoughts are decreasing, you are getting better...

...end of story.

Long-Term Doesn't Mean Incurable

I read a Facebook comment recently from a man in response to a woman who had found meditation had cured her insomnia. The comment was very dismissive, saying something along the lines of 'If she managed to cure insomnia with meditation then she can't really have had proper insomnia in the first place.' This has to be one of the strongest cases of 'insomnia is my identity' I have ever come across. So wedded was this man to the idea that his insomnia was real, was medical, was incurable, that he could not allow the possibility that someone else had overcome it so easily.

The funny thing is, in my experience, there is no direct correlation at all between the severity of a problem, and how difficult it is to overcome.

Indeed, sometimes those who have suffered for decades are the ones to make the fastest recovery.

The Endless Search

Do you harbour hopes that any moment now, doctors will come up with a new medication which actually *works?* Do your ears prick up whenever you hear of a brand new treatment on the market? Do you secretly ask yourself 'could *this* finally be the answer?'

Are you still hoping, wondering, searching for the elusive miracle 'cure for insomnia'?

You will never find it...If you are looking for the cure outside of your thoughts, behaviours and beliefs, then you are looking in the wrong place.

It took 15 years for me to accept this. Please don't be as stubborn as I was.

Hooray for Bad Nights

It may sound paradoxical, but bad nights can be a *blessing* if you respond to them well.

If you can have a really bad night of sleep but still remain positive, buoyant and full of hope, this can add infinitely more to your long term recovery than a great night of sleep.

More than anything, it is successful handling of these occasional bad nights and bad stretches which will indicate just how much better you really are.

From Night Owl to Early Bird

Not a morning person? Are you a 'night owl'? That's exactly what I once thought. Because I had hated getting up for school, I avoided doing 'proper' jobs for years. I despised mornings so much I honestly thought it would be impossible for me ever to get to work on time.

I can't believe how all this has changed. Now I love getting up early. I go out and get my morning coffee from a local café and like to be their first customer of the day. It gives me a real kick knowing I'm up and about while half the country is still in bed. It feels like I'm one step ahead of the world, in control and relaxed.

If you wish you could get up earlier, don't hide behind the 'not a morning person' label. It really doesn't mean anything.

I went from confirmed 'night owl' to 'early bird'. If I can learn to love early mornings, anyone can!

Tackle the Whole, not Just the Parts

Strange though it may seem, sleeping badly is only one small part of insomnia. Other aspects include obsessive negative thinking, worrying, talking about your problem, calling yourself an insomniac, continually researching cures and creating silly routines and rituals. All these things go to make up the entire package we call 'chronic insomnia.'

This is why a couple of good nights are rarely enough to wipe out the problem.

So, if you sleep well one night, but continue with all these other insomnia behaviours, don't be surprised when the problem reappears.

And even if you don't sleep, as long as you are not indulging in these other parts of the package, *you will still be getting better.*

All Negativity, or Just Some Negativity?

I was recently asked the following question:

"Do *all* negative thoughts affect sleep, or just those negative thoughts about sleep itself?"

For some people, a general negativity may be the problem. Many find that the more negative and depressed they are, the worse they sleep.

But for others, the opposite is true. Some depressed people sleep way more than usual. Plus, in my experience, some of the most positive, high-achievers are those with the worst insomnia.

So, when it comes to sleep, the thoughts to work on are definitely those which are most to do with sleep.

Having said that, why not banish those other negative thoughts anyway and sort the rest of your life out too

Advice for Complete Newbies

Sometimes I get asked for advice by a friend who has suffered with poor sleep for a few days, or perhaps a week. But what *is* the best advice for dealing with a brand new sleep problem?

On the one hand, it's important to nip things in the bud as quickly as possible before fear and habit kick in. But on the other, get it wrong and there could be a much greater problem.

Typically, when someone is only just starting out, I give them very, *very* basic sleep hygiene advice, tell them to get some exercise, back away slowly and *shut up*. I don't call a few days later to ask how they are sleeping. I don't email extra bits of advice. I don't even hand them a copy of my book.

Actually, I pretty much ignore them.

I'm sure some people are surprised at my apparent lack of interest in their fledgling sleep problems. But I can't tell them not to worry. I can't tell them that fear feeds insomnia, that if they pay too much attention to it, things could get much, much worse. That would be giving them chronic insomnia on a plate.

On the other hand, this 'playing the whole thing down' technique *works* every time.

Learn from My Mistakes

I have heard today from Laura, a new insomniac who was so terrified by my story at the start of *The Effortless Sleep Method* she now fears getting worse. She fears the same fate will befall her and she will suffer for as long as I did.

Remember, I am an example of what happens when you get it wrong, and wrong, and wrong...for 15 years.

If you don't want to end up with the same story, do what I *do*, not what I *did*, simple as that.

Learn from my mistakes; don't repeat them.

Rushing not Required

Patience … patience … patience …

Don't become impatient with your rate of recovery. Some people get over their insomnia very quickly, but others take much longer. And the really ironic thing is, the more you stress about how long it's taking, the longer it takes.

If you are being impatient with your progress it means you are, to some extent, still focussing on what is *wrong* more than what is *right*.

So, try to accept that wherever you are in your recovery is *just right for you.* Cultivate this attitude more fully and I promise you: *full recovery will come much sooner*.

So let recovery takes as long as it needs, *not* because full recovery necessarily takes a long time, but because letting it takes its time will result in a quicker recovery!

No Overnight Fixes

Do you really think that getting over your insomnia will involve your never again missing a night? Do you think you will never again have a negative thought or a twinge of fear? Don't imagine for one second that the sudden occurrence of one of these things mean you aren't getting better.

No-one makes a complete and full recovery overnight. I certainly didn't. It was probably a year before I was fully, and I mean *fully*, recovered.

And I'm still getting better now.

Hooray for Fear

If the fear of missing sleep is proving difficult to shake off, try neutralising this fear in the following way ...

Imagine in detail all the ways in which a bad night is actually a *good* thing. It could be that because you haven't slept, you will be able to take it easy today. It could be that you will have a chance to show just how well you can cope. It could be that you will have a chance to fully face the problem, to examine your own thoughts and feelings. It could be that you will be able to reward yourself with a special breakfast!

It doesn't matter how reasonable or true it sounds. We are just trying to dissolve, weaken and neutralise a little of that fear, to make that panicky reaction a little less panicky.

Welcome the fear in, and you can watch it evaporate.

Don't Get Caught
on a Wild Goose Chase

I remember when I was convinced that my insomnia was caused by some kind of self-sabotage mechanism. I spent years and thousands of pounds inquiring into, analysing, therapising, treating my self-sabotage mechanism.

I also remember when I was convinced that my insomnia was a control issue. I was (and still am) a bit of a control freak. I spent years and thousands of pounds inquiring into, analysing, therapising, treating my control issue.

But when I had dealt with that issue, I remember instead thinking it was a fear issue, a fear of sleep, a sleep phobia. I spent years and thousands of pounds inquiring into, analysing, therapising...

...you get the message.

Midnight Nature Calls

I do 'go on' about getting out of bed when you can't sleep, going to another room and totally changing your focus. I even think it helps to wake yourself up to a certain extent, to start that falling asleep process all over again.

But please understand that this does *not* apply to those times when you wake up in the night needing the toilet, or to get a drink of water, or to close a rattling window. In those instances, it's best to rouse yourself as little as possible, even if it means feeling your way to the bathroom in the dark like a sleepy ghost. Try to stay in that dreamy, drowsy place as you do whatever you have to.

Get this right, and eventually you'll find yourself able to get up and get a drink, close the window or answer the call of nature literally, in your sleep.

Victims and Villains

Sometimes people complain to me: 'Sasha, why do you always blame the victim?'

I don't remember ever actually using the word 'blame' but let's take a closer look at this.

If 'blame' means you have done something bad, stupid, that you should be punished, that you *deserve* insomnia, then *no*, you are not to blame at all.

But if it means keeping appalling sleep hygiene in a desperate attempt to get some rest, popping pills because you won't risk a night without them, and talking obsessively about your problem because it fills your every thought and has taken over your life …

… then yes, you are to blame for your insomnia.

But this has *nothing* to do with whether you deserve it, because no one *ever* deserves insomnia.

The whole idea of 'blaming the victim' presupposes that we are directing attention away from the true culprit – the true criminal, the true villain. But who is the villain here? There isn't one. There are only circumstances, and there is you.

The good news is that both of these things are, to some extent, within your control. Go looking for the villain of the piece and there's a good chance you'll be looking forever.

Don't Blame Me

You know what? Let's stop this talk of 'victims'. And let's stop this 'Sasha just blames the victim' nonsense. What a discouraging notion is 'victim'? It means utter disempowerment, utter helplessness. It means 'someone else did this to me, and *they* are the ones who need to put it right, not me.' Think this way, and you'll stay in that disempowered, helpless state for the rest of your life.

By taking *responsibility* for your own recovery (no matter how unfair that may seem) you *take control*. And in taking back your control, you suddenly have every chance of beating this thing.

Blame the victim? Give it a rest! It's *this sort of talk* that creates victims in the first place.

Taming Wild Fluctuations

Lily wrote to me recently to ask if it was normal to have changing sleep habits. She was surprised to hear that these types of fluctuations are actually very common.

Sleep habits seem to go through 'phases'. Sometimes I am able to sleep solidly until morning without even waking once. This will go on for some weeks, but then the pattern will change and I will wake up several times every night. Sometimes I can go through a period of really light sleep for a week or so, or with taking over an hour to fall asleep.

And I hear the same stories from everyone.

The good news is that the opposite can also happen - you can go through a period of absolutely brilliant sleep for a few weeks, for no apparent reason at all!

It really helps to try to view every good night as the beginning of one of these brilliant stretches. Why not try this yourself?

Just try thinking the following:

'Perhaps *tonight* will be the new best sleep of my life'.

The Season of Snuffles

It's flu season!

With so many colds about, there are a lot of snuffly snorers around at the moment, keeping their partners awake with coughing, spluttering, fidgeting and nose-blowing.

Now, if you are kept awake by loud snores, coughs or other fluey disturbances, don't worry too much about this being indicative of insomnia returning. Not sleeping through your partner's loud snoring is not insomnia any more than not sleeping through torture is insomnia!

If you have the luxury, it's fine to escape to the spare room for now!

Listen to Your Body

Do you find yourself nodding off in front of the television at 9.30, only to find yourself wide awake at midnight? Do you also find that you feel tired even though you are getting a decent amount of sleep?

If so, try this little trick. Try shifting your whole block of sleep forward or back by an hour or more. If you are currently sleeping 1am- 8.30, try shifting the time to 12.30- 7.30, or even to 11.30-6.30.

You may find you always feel better if you go to bed before 11 or 12. Leave it too late and you may find you feel rough no matter how much sleep you get. If I ever get into a habit of sleeping until after 8.30 or 9, I always feel exhausted all day, even when I have slept like a log.

There are a lot of theories about why this is so. I just prefer to think many of us have an inbuilt clock which determines when we find it easier and best to sleep.

This move is not likely to cure insomnia, but a little experimentation could lead to a big improvement in how you feel.

'Clinically Tested'
Doesn't Mean Effective

Still thinking a pill will cure you? Worried my method hasn't been 'clinically tested' in double-blind randomised trials?

I just don't understand why some people are happy to swallow every 'clinically-tested' chemical their doctor has been persuaded to prescribe by a pharmaceutical giant, despite suffering horrible side-effects and no improvement in their sleep...

...while these same people are often the most resistant to following a bit of common sense advice about changing sleep behaviours and associated thoughts because this evidence is merely 'anecdotal'.

Clinically speaking, I don't think anyone has ever *cured* chronic insomnia with sleeping pills, not *ever*.

Anecdotally speaking, thousands, maybe millions, have cured their insomnia with thought and behaviour modification.

What more proof do you need?

It Happens to the Best of Us

You've heard me talk before of my son, Robin, who has seemingly endless energy and optimism, is able to miss nights through choice, without thinking about it, and who sleeps like a baby. In fact, Robin sleeps so deeply he needs to set two or three alarm clocks to wake him in the morning. And he must place them on the other side of the bedroom to *force* himself out of bed!

Well, last night, it turns out he had real difficulties sleeping. He missed a whole night *for no reason whatsoever*. Yes, it happens to all of us, even the very best sleepers.

But, because this missed night has no significance whatsoever, he will just brush it off. And because he allows it no significance, Robin's 'insomnia' will last precisely *one night*.

It's Just a Bad Patch

As far as I'm concerned, if you are following the promises, there *are* no relapses.

But there are certainly bad patches. Everyone experiences them, even me.

If you are a chronic insomniac, these bad patches take on a bigger significance, and because of this, they may last little longer. Other than that, there is *no difference* between the bad patch of a good sleeper and the bad patch of bad sleeper.

So please, learn to stop thinking in terms of relapses, of setbacks. Learn to think in terms of 'a bad patch'. Because a bad patch has a finite duration, a bad patch always, *always* comes to an end.

A *relapse,* on the other hand, has no foreseeable end point. So let's banish talk of relapses!

One, Two, Insomnia

Fretting and worrying about one night turns one night into two nights.

Fretting and worrying about two nights turns two nights into a bad stretch.

Fretting and worrying about a bad stretch turns a bad stretch into insomnia.

It really is that simple…

On Sleeping Through the Night

Do you wish you could sleep right through the night, just like all normal sleepers do? Well, it may surprise you to know that most people wake almost every night to use the toilet, to have a drink or just for no reason at all.

But there is no need to panic and remain awake for ages.

When you wake, instead of panicking, just think to yourself:

Oh goody, it's still dark. That means I have loads of lovely sleep left.

And snuggle back into bed with a smile on your face, to start the delicious 'falling-asleep' process all over again.

It just takes a bit of practise, before your mind starts thinking this way naturally.

You Can't Pick and Choose

I know I've talked about this before, but I getting so many letters all on the same subject, I thought I had better revisit.

People are writing to ask why the method hasn't worked for them. Usually, they will be keeping good sleep hygiene but will often still be researching, complaining, and completely putting their insomnia before everything.

If you write to me to tell me the method isn't working, and then go on to give me a lengthy account of the history of your problem, how much you are suffering and how much worse and different it seems to all the others you hear about, and how the positive thinking doesn't work for you... *then you aren't following the method at all.*

Use Less Sleep to Create More Sleep

When you fear a bad patch is setting in, often the best thing to do is simply implement Promise 1 – *spend less time in bed* – a little more strictly.

Next time you get a couple of poor nights, and there is nothing obvious to explain them (like illness or extreme stress), the first thing you should always try is just to reduce your time spent in bed by half an hour or so. The resulting extra little bit of sleepiness is often just enough to give you a better night. It sounds too simple, but this one little trick can sometimes nip things in the bud, preventing a bad night from becoming a bad stretch of nights.

Obsessing About the Way You Feel

If you focus hard enough on what's wrong with the way you are feeling, you are bound to end up feeling something bad.

You may also find that even after a *good* night you *still* find yourself checking the way you are feeling. 'Am I tired, could I feel better, shall I meditate, do I need more coffee, should I attempt a nap?' And the funny thing is, by the evening, you will often feel almost as bad as when you have missed sleep!

Stop wasting time focussing on the way you feel, and get on with your life. You'll discover that lack of sleep doesn't actually feel so bad when you don't spend so much time thinking about it.

You Booze, You Lose

In *small* quantities, alcohol *can* be used as a 'reward' at the end of the day, encouraging a feeling of drowsy well-being conducive to good sleep.

But drink yourself into a stupor, and you'll find that alcohol dehydrates, depresses and can cause you to waken too early in the morning with a full bladder, an adrenaline rush and a pounding heart as the chemicals leave your bloodstream.

I'm not against the drinking of alcohol *per se* (I'm British, after all!) But using alcohol *as a sleep aid* can be a really bad idea.

(And this is all before we've even got to the hangover...)

No Need to Get Heated

Many people find it almost impossible to sleep if they are too cold.

Getting warm, comfy and cosy in bed is important, particularly in the first few minutes of lying down. You don't want to be spending those first few vital minutes in bed trying to warm up.

But strangely, this does *not* mean having a toasty warm room. Research shows that most people sleep best in a warm bed but in a cool, or even *cold* room. So turn off the heating in the bedroom at night, pile up the blankets and wear fluffy pyjamas.

Or even treat yourself to that most wonderful of inventions - an electric blanket! I challenge anyone not to look forward to going to bed in the winter when an electric blanket is waiting for them.

The Power of Attention

I have been prone to bouts of depression over the years, usually only lasting a few days. But in the last couple of years or so, these bouts seemed to be growing in frequency and severity, sometimes lasting weeks. It was becoming disabling and was quite scary. Everyone around me was keen to tell me it was just 'hormones', and was something I would have to get used to.

But I wasn't willing to accept this.

I decided to walk my own talk and apply my principles to the depression. I simply ignored it, did my utmost not to let a bad mood take hold (although this felt impossible at first), distracted myself, got loads of exercise, and got on with my day. I also started 'telling a new story' – that my mood was excellent these days, that life seemed to be getting better and better, that life was *perfect*. I seized life with both hands and got on with things.

It worked far better than I ever expected. It's been around six months now and I've hardly experienced a bad mood, let alone a depression! For the first time in decades, I have been experiencing frequent moments of what can only be described as pure 'joy'…

… and all that has really changed is *the focus of my attention*.

Night Time Nature Calls

Many people have an obsessional need to visit the toilet whenever they wake up in the night, whether they need it or not. It can then be difficult for them get back to sleep.

In this particular case, the waking is usually just another habit – the result of the getting up to use the toilet so often. Your body gets so used to the pattern, that it wakes you in anticipation of the getting up.

If you have this problem (and your doctor has told you there is absolutely no underlying physical or medical reason for it) the best thing you can do is to spend a few nights denying yourself these toilet visits. This may interfere with sleep for a night or two, but it won't be long before your body starts to 'notice' that you are no longer getting out of bed. It will then gradually stop bothering to wake you and the association will break.

Of course, if you *really* need to go, then go!

Thinking and Sleeping, and Thinking

I have had a real spate of people writing to me all saying the same thing. 'I'm getting better, but sometimes I can't stop the negative thoughts.'

Take comfort in this... thinking is always slow to catch up. Those negative thoughts always seem to linger long after the sleep has otherwise picked up. By focussing on the lack of progress as a problem in its own right, you actually slow down this 'catching-up' process. Focus instead on how less often these thoughts are occurring, on how much better you sleep despite the thoughts. You can even smile at them, knowing their days are numbered.

Let them be, don't give them any power, and watch them slowly fade.

Turn Mistakes into Triumphs

If you make a mistake by lying in way past your getting-up time, fall asleep on public transport or accidentally take an unplanned nap on the sofa, don't beat yourself up about it.

While these activities are not to be encouraged, at least in the early days, use these opportunities to congratulate yourself on how easily sleep is coming to you these days, how deeply you are sleeping in the morning, or how relaxed you must be to nod off without meaning to.

In fact, as Christina, one of my clients reminded me this morning, why not make these experiences into a shiny new safety thought?

How Not to Take a Nap

A couple of people have asked the same question this week: When that irresistible sleepiness comes over you, either in the afternoon or early evening in front of the television, how do you resist the temptation to take a quick nap?

The answer isn't any great mystery. You do something, *anything* which makes it impossible to sleep. Go outside and feel the air on your face, make a cup of tea, have a non-sugary snack, take a shower…anything which will wake you up a bit or prevent you from sleeping. That sleepy feeling will always pass eventually.

And you won't have to do this every day for the rest of your life – it's just until your sleeping patterns normalise and that afternoon nap desire will become a thing of the past.

Zen and the Art of Falling Asleep

Lots of people have success with the 'doing nothing' technique I mention in *The Effortless Sleep Method*, and want to know more about it.

There is no real documentation about this technique (if it can be called a technique at all). It's something I fell upon while practising Zen meditation (sometimes referred to as 'the art of doing nothing').

The main difference between Zen and 'doing nothing' is this: the main purpose of my 'doing nothing' technique is to fall asleep, whereas the purpose of Zen is to become even more aware, even more 'awake'.

But don't let this 'awakening' effect put you off meditation. Besides the myriad of positive other effects, *falling asleep* whilst meditating is one of the biggest problems for new practitioners.

Hardly surprising, really. Because meditation can be both relaxing *and* boring!

Mysterious Symptoms

Do you suffer with sore itchy eyes, unexplained aches, tickles flutters or other inexplicable symptoms even though your doctor tells you there's nothing wrong?

This is so very common. Because insomniacs tend to focus on every tiny nuance of they way they are feeling, every slight tickle, flutter or ache suddenly takes on huge significance. These sorts of symptoms always become much worse than they need to, because the more we focus on them, the worse they get. This just makes us worry more and focus on them even harder.

I'm not saying ignore worrying symptoms, but concentrating on the way you are feeling in every moment will lead you to discover all sorts of weird things going on in that magnificent and oh-so-busy body of yours.

Truth is, we *all* get funny feelings, *all* the time

Power to the Placebo

I just received an email from Tracy in New York. I get them like this occasionally...

"Your book has really helped me. But deep down I worry it's just placebo."

My reply?

"Remove the word 'just' and I would totally agree with you."

Running in the Family

Many people assume that because their mother and grandmother had sleeping problems, that they have somehow inherited the same 'genetic' disorder. This can lead to a level of hopelessness about the condition and the belief that they are broken, different and incurable.

But this is a little like thinking you have inherited smoking. Insomnia, like smoking, can be passed from parent to child as a habit. Bad habits are picked up easily, which is why insomnia often appears to run in families.

And *all* bad habits can be broken.

Just because your mother had insomnia, doesn't mean it need be a life-sentence for you.

It's Not Worth Losing Your Job Over

I often hear from people who are considering giving up their jobs because of insomnia. If this is the *only* reason you are thinking of leaving your job then *please reconsider.*

I stayed in further education, then academia, then self-employment, all in an attempt to hide away from the real world; all to avoid having to adhere to someone else's timeframe; all to avoid the risk of insomnia.

Don't do it. *It doesn't work.*

In fact, it has the opposite effect. Giving up your job could end up being a long slippery slope into basing your whole life around insomnia.

You don't want to end up where I did.

You Can Control Your Thoughts

I have seen many people get over psychological problems simply by refusing to think about them.

For the next few weeks, try this...

Whenever you think a negative thought about sleep, or a fear pops into your head, I want you to *gently,* but immediately, *change your mind* and start thinking about something, anything else. Think about what you had for lunch, a film you want to see, the colour of the bus driver's shirt, *anything.* Don't allow that negative thought any space in your head at all.

Don't try this with any deep-seated emotional issues, just with these silly, pointless negative thoughts about sleep.

Starved of attention, those pointless thoughts will eventually wither away and die.

You Don't Have to Go Cold Turkey

For many people, as soon as they I realise what the pills are really doing to them, and the effect they are having on their confidence and belief in their ability to sleep, they give them up instantly. And the first really good night's sleep without pills is always a real milestone.

But I really don't recommend you do this.

For a start, this sort of 'cold turkey' approach can be really dangerous, even fatal.

But secondly, stopping immediately is too big a jump for some people. It is likely to throw you into a panic, sabotaging your recovery and possibly undoing all the good you have so far achieved. Lots of people get into a terrible state because they rush to give up sleeping pills.

There is no point in scaring yourself, bringing on rebound insomnia, and then becoming despondent. All we need is a *little* bit of progress, a *little* improvement. So don't rush to stop.

Far better is to reduce the dose *slowly*, really slowly. If you want to cut down by half a pill a week, or quarter of a pill a *month* that's fine. Marja, one of my therapy clients, is currently cutting down by one *tiny* crumb at a time. And she gives herself a big pat on the back every time she does .

Remember, every night of even *slightly* better sleep, with even *slightly* less medication is a triumph, and is to be celebrated even if the reduction is very small indeed.

Give up your medication at whatever speed you can feel comfortable. You don't have to rush to your first milestone.

Turn Frustration to Triumph

Isn't it frustrating? Sometimes, you can be doing really well. Sleep has been great for weeks. Then, for no reason, a bad night comes along, and then another.

Disaster?

Not at all! If a bad patch comes along, just when everything was going so well, this is great news! This means it has been ages since your last bad night. Celebrate that and just look forward to the next run of good sleep. And if you keep up this attitude, you won't have long to wait.

What Are You Afraid of?

Don't ever try and 'suppress' the fear. It will only pop out and bite you at the worst possible moment. Much better is to try and 'allow' the fear to be there. Look at it full in the face, see what it has to say...

The fear itself is always worse than the thing you're afraid of.

Will Insomnia Damage Your Health?

Many people have written to me worrying about possible permanent damage to their health caused by long term insomnia.

To be honest, I think the negative effects of insomnia on long term physical health may be exaggerated. There is a lot of scaremongering in the media, telling you that getting less than eight hours sleep a night results in instant death or some other such nonsense.

These types of scare story actually have the opposite effect to the one intended by making the problem worse. I hear from a lot of people who are terrified they are threatening their health, even their very lives with sleep deprivation.

Fear is the enemy of sleep, and scaring people half to death with a bleak vision of their future health if they don't get some sleep, well…that's hardly conducive to good sleep.

And if we look to science for answers, it's hard to find any agreement on the matter. Some scientists seem to think that not getting enough sleep can lower your immune system, and lead to a greater incidence of serious illness. But there are also numerous studies which show that those who get less no more than five or six hours a night actually live longer than the rest of us.

For every study which tells you that getting more sleep is healthier, I can point you to another which says the opposite.

And you know, almost every day I hear from people who *fear* illness through lack of sleep. But although I hear from the most chronic insomniacs every single day, *thousands* of them, I can't remember a single person ever telling me they have become seriously ill as a result of insomnia.

Just an observation. Make of it what you will.

Crutches Aren't So Bad

Long-term insomniacs will usually have a whole host of negatively reinforcing behaviours such as taking medication, talking up the problem and compromising their lives. If using a harmless external crutch means that those more destructive behaviours can be eliminated, this can be a helpful half way stage in your recovery. I am talking about such things as earplugs, special recordings, or (and I am hearing about this more and more) sleeping in the spare room or on the sofa.

And if you want to eliminate the crutch at some point, it will be a whole lot easier to stop this one, non-destructive habit when all those other negative behaviours have been eliminated and your sleeping habits are normal and regular.

Change Your Life in 14 Days

I have challenged you before to attempt to spend one day without saying anything negative about your sleep, but you can also take this one step further.

One my favourite pieces of advice, one I like to give to really chronically negative thinkers, those who plunge into despair after every less-than-perfect night, is this...

For two weeks, you are not allowed to complain or say anything negative about your sleep, not *once.* This applies, not just to what you say to other people, but also when talking to yourself. If you do complain, you must start the fortnight all over again the following day.

For many people, this is such a massive change in behaviour that this little piece of advice alone can have a profound effect on sleep, and on the beliefs surrounding it. Martin from The Netherlands wrote to tell me following this advice has 'transformed his experience of life'.

And if you like it, you can try this on all your other negative thinking too.

How to Become an Olympian Sleeper

There is no Olympic sleeping team. There are no gold medals for being a champion sleeper. Pity really. I would have suggested we all enter ourselves.

The training? Well, that's easy. Just keep good sleep hygiene, let go of all the worrying, and then focus on becoming...not just an '*ok*' sleeper...not just a *good* sleeper...but an Olympic gold medal winning sleeper.

With your eye on *that* prize, you would be too focussed to nit-pick over tiny details of your sleep experience, you wouldn't have time to fuss over the odd missed night, and you certainly wouldn't risk losing everything by cheating and taking performance-enhancing sleeping drugs.

With sleep (but not, sadly with other sports), it really is that easy.

Turn the Fear on Its Head
(aka 'Becoming a Bully')

Like the victim who has his or her tormentor in a cage, you can bully and torment your insomnia once it is powerless. I once lived in terror of this enemy, but I have turned this fear on its head. I now taunt and tease the insomnia 'monster', just to prove how good a sleeper I have become. I set myself new challenges all the time: I decide to sleep out in the open air, or in the car, just for fun. Given a choice, I choose the noisier, smaller, less comfortable room. And sometimes I stay up all night intentionally, just to see how good I can still feel the next day.

Because I am the one in control, these things no longer hold any fear for me and every new success only boosts my confidence further.

Eventually you will turn the fear on its head, just like I have done. Once you can show total courage in the face of this fear, *only then* will you finally escape from insomnia.

It's a Bumpy Old Road

If you miss a night, it doesn't mean you got something wrong.

If lack of sleep makes you depressed, *you're normal.*

If you find it hard to control your thoughts and feelings, *join the club.*

By judging yourself for having individual issues you just add an additional layer of misery to the issues themselves. Remember, you are learning to sleep again, and this can be a bumpy road.

So be a little kinder to yourself, and realise that everything that happens is *just fine.*

On Magical Thinking

I am not an advocate of magical thinking... where all your desires miraculously pop into existence just because you think about them.

But I know this: if you tell a child it's unlovable, it becomes that. If you tell yourself you're unworthy, you become that. If you tell yourself you're fantastic, you become that.

If you tell yourself you're an insomniac…

I'll let you finish the sentence

What if You Knew
You Wouldn't Sleep?

Think about this...which of the following thoughts gives you more peace

'I may or may not sleep tonight' or

'I won't sleep tonight'?

A large part of what makes missing sleep so unpleasant is the *wondering, the internal wrangle* that precedes it, the confusion, the not-knowing: should I exercise, or drink coffee, or watch television in bed, or eat turkey and milk for dinner?

If you *knew* you wouldn't sleep tonight, for example if you were going to an all-night party, the feeling would be completely different. And bizarrely, taking off the pressure in this way can also have the effect of relaxing the mind enough to sleep.

So, there can even a perverse *comfort* in the thought 'I won't sleep tonight'

Don't Believe the Statistics

I have seen 'Insomnia' defined as the inability to fall asleep within 30 minutes more than twice a week. But only someone who is always asleep within seconds could imagine that there is necessarily something wrong with the person who takes more than 30 minutes to drop off.

Many people who consider themselves to be excellent sleepers take up to an hour or more to fall asleep at night, and certainly should not be described as insomniacs.

Don't let statistics like this scare you.

This too, Shall Pass

If you are having a really bad day, it can be difficult to find a spark of positivity or hope. I found a great quote on Facebook that I'd like to repeat here. I don't know where it comes from, or who authored it, but perhaps it will give a little comfort.

"On particularly rough days when I'm sure I can't possibly endure, I like to remind myself that my track record for getting through bad days so far is 100%, and that's pretty good."

Just remember, bad days always, *always* come to an end.

Fear of Late Nights

It is quite common that a person will stick religiously to a certain bedtime, fearing that any divergence will result in a sleepless night and a return of the bad times. Some will even avoid social events and parties that go on past their normal bedtime, for fear of interfering with sleep.

The result is that they are just as imprisoned by their insomnia as they ever were, only now by the fear of being 'up past bedtime'.

The answer is to turn this situation on its head. If you are afraid to go to events that finish past midnight, then sit up one night past midnight *and just watch TV*.

If you are afraid to be out past 2am, then stay up until 2.30am occasionally, not because of social occasions, but just for no *reason whatsoever*. Do it until it no longer feels scary. Do it until sleep comes easily. By proving to yourself that you can sleep on non-important nights, you will be much better able to sleep after those big social occasions.

PS. This advice is designed to help OK sleepers become good sleepers. It is not recommended for those who have not even begun to recover

Placebo or Nocebo?

A bit of science for you...

Placebo : the *positive* effect of a treatment or diagnosis.

Nocebo: the *negative* effect of a treatment or diagnosis.

We have all heard of the placebo effect – this is when a totally inactive treatment for a particular condition actually causes an improvement in that condition.

But you may not be aware of another newly-documented phenomenon – the *nocebo* effect. This happens when a in inactive treatment for a condition, or even the diagnosis alone, can cause a *worsening* of that condition.

So before your diagnose yourself, or accept a diagnosis of psychophysiological insomnia, genetic insomnia or any other official-sounding condition, be aware, be *very* aware of the possibility of the *nocebo* effect.

Becoming Distracted

Do you know the best way of dealing with negative thoughts? It's not to analyse them or try to work out why they are there. And it certainly isn't to become frustrated and angry with yourself over their continued presence in your life. No, the best way of dealing with negative thoughts is *distraction*.

When a negative though pops in, rather than indulging it in any way at all, much better is to get up immediately and do something, anything. Think of something else, call someone, pick up a book, go for a walk, start a conversation. This will serve instantly to drain some of the power and energy from that thought and so lessen its impact. Drain enough of its power and it will fade away and die.

Practice Makes Perfect

Don't tell me you can't change your thoughts. Don't tell me you have no control over them. Don't tell me affirmations 'don't work on you'. You *can*, you *have* and they *do*.

But after months, years or decades of habitual negative thinking, you can't just say 'I'm a great sleeper' and expect that circumstance magically to appear in your life. You have to work at it, over and over. You have to practise until it becomes the norm. *You have to make it a habit.*

On Waking Up
JUST as You Are Falling Asleep

A few people have asked me recently about this strange phenomenon of jumping into wakefulness *just* as they are about to fall asleep. They tell me it's as if they suddenly become aware of becoming unconscious when a thought pops in, or their heart 'jumps' or they feel a little rush which then sparks them into wakefulness.

What you probably don't realise is that almost every single person complains of this! This little thought or adrenaline rush is really just a symptom of high tension, low expectation and paying too much attention to your physical state. It doesn't have any great significance in the big scheme of things and it certainly doesn't require any special attention or treatment. In fact, the best thing you can do about it is nothing at all.

If you focus on this twinge, that itch, the funny feeling in your chest, that fluttery feeling, it will grow and become a problem in itself. (But always get heart palpitations checked out by a doctor!)

For those who suffer with this sudden 'jumping' into wakefulness just on the point of sleep, the very best bedtime method to use is what I call 'Doing Nothing'. The advantage of this is that when using this 'technique', sleep often comes suddenly, without any memory of having become drowsy. With no conscious awareness of falling asleep, there will be no sudden jump, no heart-flip, no adrenaline rush, and a better chance of falling asleep.

Out of the Blue

It's frustrating, isn't it? Just when things are going really well, just when you think you have turned a corner, a bad night or two comes along out of the blue.

What went wrong? What has stopped working?

When this happens please *don't* waste any time focussing on those bad nights. Don't imagine that you have done something wrong, or that something has stopped working. This will happen again and again before you are fully recovered and should not surprise you.

Instead, decide to show the world just how great a day you can have, even after a bad night. And then... just look forward to the next little bit of good sleep.

Keep up this attitude and that next good night won't be far away.

No Compromises

Dear Friends, these are some questions I have been asked recently, and their answers...

Q: 'Should I cancel my birthday party in case I don't sleep the night before?'
A: *No*
Q: 'Should I put off having a family until I am better?'
A: *No*
Q: 'Should I get a job with more flexible hours?'
A: No

Every compromise to insomnia, reinforces insomnia.

Doing What You Know

Do you have a healthy interest in current sleep research?

While reading, you will probably learn a lot about how big a problem insomnia is, you will learn that there are different types of insomniacs, you will hear about new medications, and trials on various gadgets. And you will be told again and again the coffee and tea can keep you awake. But how often do you actually learn anything *really* important regarding overcoming insomnia? Have you ever picked up a piece of information which actually enabled *you personally* to sleep?

Overcoming insomnia is not about assimilating more and more knowledge. It does not involve doing more painstaking research online. It does not involve subscribing to scientific sleep journals. It involves carrying out instructions, not just reading them. It involves following advice, not just listening. Otherwise, this all just becomes another insomnia-reinforcing behaviour.

Overcoming insomnia is not an intellectual process. It is an *experiential* process.

Maybe that interest in sleep research isn't so healthy.

What to Do Tonight

Are you are wondering what to do tonight to give yourself the best chance of sleeping well? Are you trying to decide on the preparation, the routine, and the sleep aids you will use to make sure you sleep? If so, *stop.*

Just consider for a moment: what does a normal good sleeper do in preparation for bed? *Then do that.* How does a normal good sleeper think in preparation for bed? *Then try to think like that.*

Good sleepers don't have elaborate routines or use multiple sleep aids. Good sleepers may have a bath, watch some television, have a hot drink…not 'to make them sleep' but *because they enjoy it.* Good sleepers go to bed when tired. And good sleepers gives no thought to whether or not they will sleep.

Just try nudging yourself slightly in the direction of thinking, being and doing things *like a normal good sleeper.*

Try, Try, Try

Are you working really, really hard to get to the stage of not caring about whether or not you sleep? Are you trying your hardest to stop seeing sleep as so important? Are you doing everything you can to forget all about insomnia?

Think about it…if you are trying really hard not to care about missing sleep, *then you must still really care about missing sleep.*

If you are trying really hard not to see sleep as important, *it must still be really important to you.*

And the harder you try to forget about insomnia, *the longer it stays in your thoughts.*

So, just stop trying so hard.

And don't *ever* give yourself a hard time for not being at the correct state of mind yet. It will come. The best way to achieve this general state of 'take-it-or-leave-it' is not to try to change anything, not to focus on sleep at all. The best way to achieve this state is to get out into the world and get on with your life.

Put sleep on the back burner, just like a normal good sleeper does.

Who Wants to Be a Millionaire?

Have you heard the saying 'talk like a millionaire, think like a millionaire, act like a millionaire and you'll become a millionaire'?

Well, good luck with that… Because while a positive attitude may help, actually becoming a millionaire isn't *entirely* within our control. It depends, to some extent, upon circumstances, people and events which we cannot directly influence.

However, becoming a good sleeper is *entirely* within your control. It does not depend on outside forces, what other people think or do. It's just about you, your habits and your behaviours.

I promise you this…think, talk and act like a good sleeper and you *will* become one.

Dilemmas in Being Normal

This is only for those of you who have seen great progress and are now looking to move past insomnia, to put this all behind you and get back to having a 'normal life'. This means paying less attention to those things you currently do to help your sleep. At some point, the strict sleep hygiene needs to lessen, all the insomnia paraphernalia needs to be thrown out; you should even stop reading my books and unsubscribe from my emails.

But Joyce, one of my therapy clients, has now found herself in a dilemma over this. Should she even be *doing* the meditation? Should she be doing positive affirmations? Should she still be exercising, relaxing, staying positive? Should she try that new wonder supplement her friend mentioned? Or will all these things just reinforce her insomnia? After all, these could all be viewed as reminders of her old problem, indications that she isn't moving on, that she isn't putting it all behind her, that she isn't forgetting at all.

The answer to all of you in a similar situation is this: once you have really improved, it's absolutely fine to keep doing any and all of these things *if you enjoy them.* Do meditation because it will improve your life in a myriad of ways. If you enjoy affirmations, keep doing them but don't make them about sleep. Keep exercising because its benefits go way beyond improving sleep. Take the new supplement, as it may help you in other areas of health.

But don't do, take or practise anything 'because you have insomnia'.

Can you see the difference? If you are doing it 'for insomnia' you are reinforcing the problem. If you are doing it for other reasons (even though one happy side effect might also be an improvement in sleep) it's absolutely fine.

Building New Memories

I still remember the first time I arranged a whole weekend's activities for myself and my friends. This was something which once would have struck terror into my insomniac mind.

The night before the weekend I relaxed into my 'safety thought'

I've slept before on a high pressure night, I can do it again.

I slept fine the whole weekend, and during the day, I was having too good a time to worry or care about how I was feeling.

I celebrated this weekend for months. I thought of the occasion whenever I could and smiled at the memory.

I know it feels that you'll never be able to stop the negative thoughts that currently plague your mind. But as you improve, good memories like this will increase, gradually replacing all those nightmarish thoughts and recollections of sleepless nights and hellish days.

Soon, you won't even have to work hard on focussing on the positive, because positive will be all there is.

How to Speed Things Up

Many people ask how long they should expect to wait it until they *fully* recover. They often wonder whether their recovery is taking more or less time than usual, and whether it is progressing 'normally'. And they often want to know how they can speed things up.

It's a horrible irony but asking these sorts of questions only serves to push your full recovery further away. You will only be completely over your insomnia when you have stopped wondering, stopped questioning, stopped *thinking about insomnia*. I want you to forget about insomnia, to put it firmly in the past. And this can't happen while you are still questioning how fast your recovery is progressing.

If you really want to speed things up, you need to stop questioning, stop wondering, and just get on with your life.

Those who manage to do this successfully find insomnia slipping out of their lives without their even noticing.

Take the Challenge

If you want to become a really good sleeper, a brilliant sleeper, you need to start challenging yourself. You need to start doing the scary things which might mess with your sleep - the sorts of things that really amazing sleepers do without thinking. When they go well, these are the sorts of things that rocket your self-belief to new levels.

But be warned: these things might also well interfere with your sleep, resulting with a few bad nights the first time you attempt them. When you don't mind whether or not this happens, *only then* will you be ready to attempt your first challenge.

And the great thing is – if your sleep does suffer, you can blame the toughness of the challenge, not yourself.

Just Do It

Think of something that you would love to do, that you *could* do, that you *would* do... if only you didn't have a sleeping problem.

And then *do it!*

By taking control of your life in this way, you actually weaken your insomnia. Don't let insomnia dictate what you can and cannot do. Show a strong face to insomnia, refuse to be dominated by it.

Then watch and smile as it backs slowly away.

Remember, Remember...

Do you ever remember having a really good day, even when you hadn't slept well?

Do you ever remember having a really *bad* day, even though you had?

It's important to recognise that good and bad days just happen. There is no necessary correlation here. You can often have a really bad day, even though you slept fine.

And... you can have some of the best days of your life, having had no sleep at all.

Looking for Evidence.

'Telling a new story' can take many forms. One of the very best ways to tell a new positive story about your sleep is to look for evidence that it's true.

Imagine you are a scientist, trying to prove a theory. Imagine you are under immense pressure to come out with a certain conclusion. In these circumstances, you are extra alert to all evidence in favour of that conclusion, perhaps exaggerating its existence or credibility.

At the same time, you may be tempted to gloss over those anomalies, those odd errant results to the contrary, those instances here and there that suggest your theory is wrong.

Can you take this same attitude towards your sleep? Be on the lookout for every positive outcome, while glossing over the negatives, explaining them away, or just plain ignoring them.

This is a fabulously effective way of making your new story come true.

A Gift from the Sleep Angels

A time-traveller, or an angel, or a psychic (or someone who means something to you) visits you at breakfast with the gift of some important news:

Today is going to be the best day of your life.

The messenger then leaves you.

How would you go about your day, having received this news? Undoubtedly, you would walk around as if on a cloud, happy, expectant, absolutely relaxed and accepting of whatever came along.

Because after all, today is going to be the best day of your life! You would focus on all the good things that occurred, and bad things, if they turned up, would seem unimportant.

By the end of the day, you have had a *great day,* one in which the world just seemed sunnier, the atmosphere lighter, colours brighter. The day did turn out to be a good one, simply by virtue of your being told this information.

But…as you prepare for bed you realise: that was a good day, but it wasn't the *best ever.*

What went wrong?

At that point, the psychic/angel/time-traveller appears again with some different news: they made up the business about the 'best day ever'.

All of the goodness you saw in this day was of your own making; it was down to your own outlook, your own expectations, your own 'letting everything be okay'.

You did that…

And their *actual* gift to you…?

It is this knowledge: you can make every day as good as this one, or better, by simply setting out with the same expectations.

Sick of Me Yet?

Eventually, you'll find yourself thinking: 'I've had enough of hearing from Sasha. All she does is remind me of a problem I once had. I think I'm better off without her.'

When this happens to you, I'll know my work is done.

You will never truly be over insomnia until you have stopped obsessing, stopped rule-following, stopped thinking about insomnia. To be a true ex-insomniac you need to *forget* all about insomnia. And you will only do this by stopping doing *all* those things an insomniac does. Sooner or later, you will need to stop reading about insomnia.

Sooner or later you must forget all about me, forget all about my method and get on with your life.

So if you feel that reading this book is just reminding you of a problem you used to have, or of how bad things used to be, *great* news! This just means you are naturally thinking less and less about your problem and no longer want to be reminded of it

So, I am *never* offended when someone asks to be taken off my mailing list!

The Sky's the Limit –
Because It Doesn't End with Sleep

Once you have mastered this method, you don't have to limit its application just to your sleep. You can apply these principles to other areas.

You can do this *all the time*. If you don't like some aspect of your life, start telling a new story. Pretty soon you'll start believing it, and your life will change for the better. This isn't magic, this is not 'calling on the universe'; it is subtly and effectively making a change in *you*. And if *you* are different, your life will be different.

Isa, from Norway, told me she is now very successfully tackling her panic attacks using this method (a problem I know nothing about.)

If you don't like some aspect of your life, try telling a new story, one you would like to be true. It's amazing how often life seems to fall into step with the new narrative.

The Best Is Yet to Come

I'm excited to tell you this one...!

Last night, I had without doubt, the best sleep of my entire life. It was deep, unbroken, delicious, full of the sweetest dreams, and I awoke with a smile on my face, thinking 'I have *never* slept that well'.

It's eight years after my recovery began and my sleep just gets better and better.

The best night's sleep of *your* life could be on the horizon, not just as good as before your insomnia started, but *better than you can even imagine!*

If I Were Allowed
to Say Only One Thing...

In *The Companion* I talk at a lot of *focussing on the good, while wilfully ignoring the bad.*

This sums up almost the entire positive thinking side of the method.

Insomniacs tend to notice, exaggerate and focus on the bad nights, on the remaining problems and on what is *still wrong,* often at the expense of all the good that may be going on.

You need to reverse this focus. Notice, exaggerate, relish in your new positive story. Take every little success as *proof* that your recovery is in full swing.

Become blind to the negative aspects of your problem. Gloss over, explain away, or *ignore* anything that is still 'wrong'.

Take this seriously. Be vigilant with it. It will make profound and wonderful changes to your life.

If I were only allowed to give one piece of advice to all the world's insomniacs, it would be this.

Telling Tall Stories

The story you tell about your sleep will come true, no exceptions.

So give your story the happiest ending you can think of.

Where to go from here?

Do you have questions? Are you wondering how to move on to the next stage of your recovery? Would you like to become not a good sleeper, but a *great* sleeper?

For the complete step-by-step method to curing even the most chronic insomnia, do seek out

The Effortless Sleep Method

You will find more advanced sleep wisdom and all your questions answered in Sasha Stephens' follow-up book

The Effortless Sleep Companion

Available now from Amazon, Barnes and Noble and from all good bookshops.

30296833R00111

Printed in Great
Britain
by Amazon